REDESIGN
YOUR
BODY

Authors' Previous Books

Starbodies

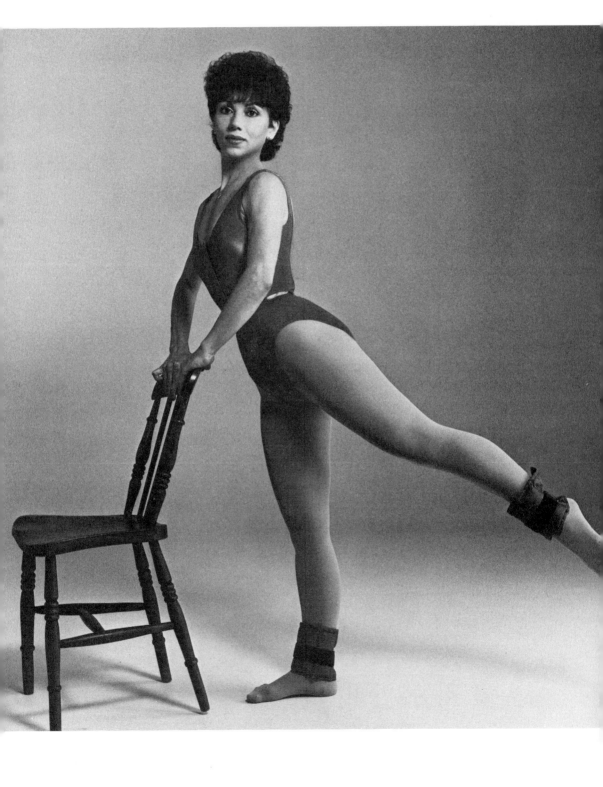

REDESIGN YOUR BODY

The 90-Day Real Body Makeover

Drs. Anita and Franco Columbu

with Paddy Calistro

E. P. DUTTON, INC./NEW YORK

Exercise photgraphs: makeup courtesy Shelly Corinne; hair courtesy Brenda Hudson; front cover makeup and hair styling courtesy Dona Desmond. Cover and exercise photographs © 1984 by Robert Gardner.

Published in the United States by E. P. Dutton, Inc.
2 Park Avenue, New York, N.Y. 10016

Library of Congress Catalog Card Number: 84–73333

ISBN: 0-525-24290-2
Published simultaneously in Canada by Fitzhenry & Whiteside, Limited, Toronto.

10 9 8 7 6 5 4 3 2 1

First Edition

To Every Woman Who Wants to Redesign Her Body

This book is your blueprint.

Your mind is the designer.

Your body is the structure.

You are the power.

CONTENTS

PREFACE

Doesn't everyone like success stories? I know I do. This book is all about success. On the following pages you'll see six women who were ready to succeed, and what they accomplished in just 90 days. By allowing themselves to become what they always wanted to be, to look the way they always wanted to look, and to feel the way they always wanted to feel, these women have not only redesigned their bodies—they've redesigned their lives. You'll read about their successes, and about how they felt during the process. Changing their appearances wasn't the easiest thing they've ever done, but all of them agree that it wasn't the hardest, either. And their efforts were richly rewarded. They look and feel beautiful. They can now live their lives at their best.

We all reach those turning points—the times in our lives when we decide to change everything for the better. The day I started to weight train was my turning point.

I had been overweight most of my life; it was a constant battle to lose. Just after college I went to California in search of ways to get my body in shape. I tried the whole gamut of diet crazes, but none of them had lasting effects. After each new diet, I ended up a few pounds lighter, but flabbier than I had been before. Every time I went on one of those unbalanced regimes, I ended up with more body fat and less energy. I rarely exercised; I never gave myself a chance to change the design of my body. Even when I dieted myself down to 115 pounds, I still had fat legs.

I devoted several years to studying the body and how to keep it healthy. Fifteen years ago I completed chiropractic college, and went on to get my Ph.D. in nutrition. But I still had my own personal battle with weight. And being the wife of Franco Columbu—Mr. Universe, Mr. World, and Mr. Olympia all rolled into one—didn't make my relationship with my body any easier. Then came the turning point.

One night I came home from my office and asked for help from Franco—who had never complained about my saddlebag thighs and pear-shaped figure. He showed me a simple training program, and I got started. Through weeks of weight training, I changed my figure. I'm convinced that exercise is the only way to make a permanent change.

The fields of exercise, health, and nutrition are constantly evolving, so I've taken hundreds of seminars and classes to keep up-to-date on the research. I've investigated the body/mind connection—the theories of positive mental programming such as positive thinking and self-hypnosis—to study its impact on weight control. Over the years I've visited spas, ashrams, and health resorts and spoken to hundreds of overweight women. I've tested the latest diets and "wonder" foods to see which, if any, of them worked. All my research has shown that to have an ideal body there are three important keys, each of which we discuss in detail throughout this book.

1. Only exercise will reshape your body.
2. Only sound nutrition will keep your body functioning properly.
3. Only a positive mental attitude will allow you to achieve your goals.

During my 20 years of study I've analyzed my own eating patterns as well as other people's. Even those who eat a nutritionally balanced diet can overeat, and that results in excess fat. I even find myself fighting that urge during times of stress and fatigue—it's a natural reaction. But again, exercise comes to my rescue. I weight train instead of eating, and my energy level and spirits soar. My patients report the same great results—and so do the world's champion athletes.

Thanks to my training program, I'm slim and I love my body. These are the words of a formerly wide-hipped, thick-thighed woman who once wore size 16 pants. Today my body looks younger and firmer than it did 20 years ago. I wear size 3 and I weigh 110 pounds. *And* I feel terrific.

You'll read the same kinds of stories about six wonderful women in this book. I want to thank Dr. Alyse Daniel, Alison Elder, Gini Gruber, Jill Richardson, Suzette Smith, and Eleanor Sobel for sharing their stories with us. It takes guts to bare your "before" body to the public, but each of them expressed a great desire to be an inspiration. We gave them the tools with which to create their success, but it was the work and positive attitude of each that allowed exercise to become part of her life. Each redesigned her own body. They all love their success—they take pride in their accomplishments. They know, and we know, that you can do it too!

A book such as this is always a joint effort. We would like to thank Bill Whitehead, Elizabeth Saft, Nancy Etheredge, Jeanne Conklin, Jacquelyn Reid, Lydia Fragomeni, Shelly Corinne, Brenda Hudson, the Santa Monica Bodybuilding Center, Scott McAuley, Kathryn Welker, Maureen and Eric Lasher, and especially Barbara Friedman and photographer Robert Gardner for their important contributions to *Redesign Your Body*.

Dr. Anita Columbu
Los Angeles, April 1984

REDESIGN
YOUR
BODY

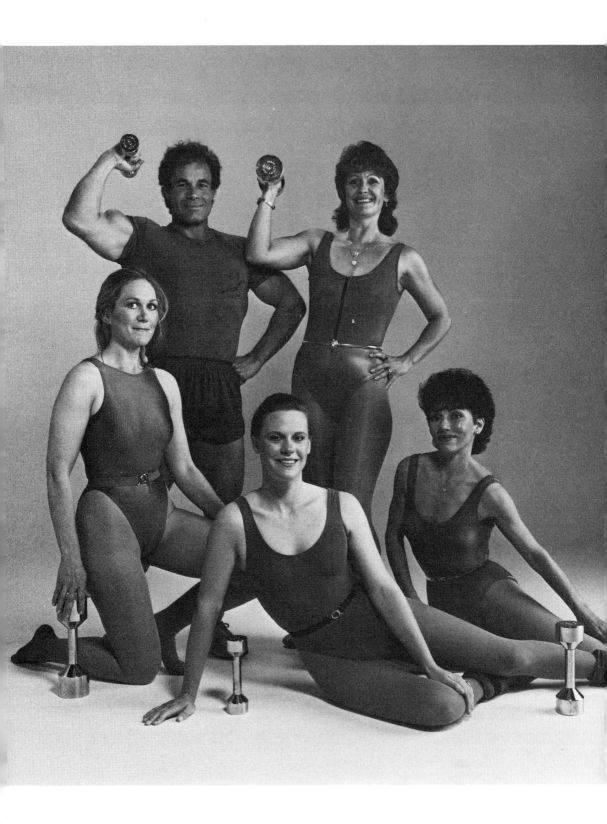

1

REDESIGN YOUR BODY

Before you start reading this book, take a moment to visualize the body you have always wanted—the way you'd look if you were in the best possible shape. Perhaps you see trimmer thighs, a slim waist, a flat stomach, rounder breasts, a hint of contour on your upper arm, or a curvier rear end. Close your eyes and picture your dream body. Keep that mental image; hold on to it for as long as you can. You are visualizing your new body—the body you *will* achieve in less time than you ever thought possible.

Have you spent too many days of your life trying to diet away those extra inches, only to realize that dieting won't do it? Have you concluded that if your body is shaped like a pear, going on a drastic diet will only make you look like a smaller pear? Have you resolved to find an *effective* way to get rid of flab and those extra pounds? If you've answered yes to any one of these questions, you're ready to accept the permanent answer to your problems.

If you've been dieting off and on for years, you've already learned one thing: Dieting can actually make you *gain* weight. Each time you cut down drastically on calories, your body adjusts to the shock. Your metabolism—the rate at which your body burns calories for energy—naturally slows down, making it increasingly more difficult to lose weight, even on just a few hundred calories. That's why most dieters reach those depressing plateaus where weight loss stops. Then, when you return to normal eating, the lower metabolism can't process the new load of calories as quickly, and you gain weight—often as much as 10 percent more than you lost. Your slower metabolism is burning fewer and fewer calories, which means you must eat less just to maintain your weight loss. That vicious circle has to be broken.

One sure way to lose weight is to eat less and *also* speed up the metabolism through exercise. Another effective way is to increase the amount of regular exercise you do without modifying the diet. In either case, exercise is the key because it helps suppress the appetite and increases the resting metabolic rate anywhere from 10 to 25 percent. But to reduce problem areas on the body, exercise must burn calories *and* trim those bulges.

To burn calories efficiently and rapidly, an exercise must be aerobic. That is, it must raise the pulse to your maximum rate (see page 144). Twelve minutes of this vigorous activity and a gradual cool-down provide a beneficial aerobic workout.

The answer is weight training—the only form of exercise that is completely aerobic *and* attacks the spot deposits of stubborn fat that camouflage your naturally beautiful body. Ideally, the female form should be composed of 20 to 25 percent body fat, but the average American woman's body is between 30 and 40 percent fat, with much of the excess localized at the stomach, hips, thighs, and derrière. Since even underweight women can have proportionately too much body fat, unsightly bulges may appear and make any woman look fatter than she actually is. By using highly concentrated energy, weight training depletes stored fat deposits and develops the body's lean muscle.

Since a pound of muscle is five times smaller in volume than a pound of fat, imagine how quickly the inches disappear!

All the women photographed in this book were displeased with the way they looked when we first met them. But there was hope: All of them were ready to take control of their bodies in order to see themselves finally looking their best.

We developed an individualized program for each of our models. The women made some very specific demands, and we listened: They wanted a program that was enjoyable, effective, and that didn't disrupt their lives—a program they could stick with. None of our models exercised more than 2 hours each day; most exercised far less. But all of them were highly motivated and ready for a complete transformation.

Almost immediately they found they'd developed increased firmness and an overall feeling of strength and well-being. All of them reported sounder sleep and less fatigue. Their spirits rose when we got out the tape measures: inches were falling off. Gini showed a 4½-inch loss from her abdomen in just 4 weeks. Jill's hips shrank 3 inches in 4 weeks too. All the women showed rapid results—the best incentive to keep going. They kept training, and they're still training. They tell us that lifting weights has become a way of life. "It frees me to eat whatever I want, whenever I want," explains Alison. "I know I'll never get out of shape again."

As you look at the "after" pictures of our models, you'll see that none of them developed a muscle-bound, unfeminine figure—their hormones didn't let that happen. Although strength can increase by as much as 50 percent, only minimal changes in the size of women's muscles occur during weight training. Testosterone, the predominant male hormone responsible for Mr. Universe muscles, is very limited in the female body (only about 3 to 5 percent of the amount found in men). Without increasing testosterone levels in the body, you can't develop a masculine form.

In fact, most women become slimmer, shapelier, and more compact—more attractively feminine—through weight training. A woman who trains will look slimmer than a sedentary woman of similar weight and build. Actually, a very well-toned slim body usually weighs more than a poorly toned body; because it is much denser, muscle mass is heavier than fat mass.

When you train with weights, changes begin to appear in as few as 4 weeks. You will achieve curves where there were bulges, contours where there was shapelessness. Your chest will become fuller, although the amount of fat deposited in your breasts will decrease. The muscles supporting them will provide a younger, higher, and rounder silhouette. Your back will broaden slightly to accentuate your trimmer waist. Fat stored on the abdomen, inner thighs, outer thighs (which some people call "saddlebags"), and even those stubborn bulges around the knees will all disappear as you begin to know the meaning of "reps" and "sets" and the difference between your pectoralis and gluteus muscles.

Nobody promises that it will be easy. But we do promise that if you stick with the program for 30 days, you'll see such amazing results that you will be *determined* to see what happens in the next 30 days. By then you'll be hooked, and on your way to the perfect body you visualized when you first opened this book.

Why is weight training the fastest way to transform your body? Count the reasons:

    1. Weight training efficiently burns more calories than any other sport.
    2. Weight training is the only true spot-reducing exercise, because certain muscle groups can be isolated and worked individually.
    3. Weight training rapidly eliminates fat from the body.
    4. Weight training takes less time to condition and develop muscle than any other sport. For instance, 7 sets of squats with weights, consisting of 20 reps

each, take about 20 minutes, yet it would take an hour of running to achieve the same results.

5. Weight training is a totally aerobic exercise, even better for the heart than running. Running increases the size of the heart muscle and allows it to pump more blood, but weight training accomplishes the same thing *and* increases the thickness of the heart muscles, which makes the heart function more efficiently. By training rapidly with weights you can increase the heart rate.

6. Weight training improves muscle tone and increases muscle strength.

7. Weight training increases the energy storage capacity in the muscles.

8. Weight training is an excellent source of aerobic exercise that can be done indoors—a big plus for people housebound by inclement weather.

9. Weight training strengthens weak areas to help prevent injuries.

10. Weight training increases circulation to the skin, discourages wrinkles, and improves skin tone.

Unlike most exercise programs, weight training can be extremely varied, using many different approaches to the same end. Your workouts can vary in routine, intensity, and frequency. And you can use a variety of different equipment—everything from high-tech machines to pulleys, dumbbells, and barbells—we've even seen women achieve great results holding, instead of dumbbells, plastic bleach bottles filled with sand! (The handles make them easy to manipulate, and by hanging the bottles on the ends of a broomstick—voilà! you have an instant barbell.) You can exercise at home, at a spa, on the beach, or even in a hotel room while you're traveling. No other exercise technique is as complete or as versatile as weight training.

Properly toned muscles mean better posture, which in turn makes you look taller, slimmer, and healthier. Weight training keeps your body properly aligned. As the muscles strengthen, they hold the bones in position and assist in correct movement. Backaches, headaches, and neck aches are often a result of poor alignment and muscle control; most of these pains are alleviated as the muscles become strengthened through training. Strong muscles also contribute to good circulation, improved digestion, nerve conduction, lymph drainage, and energy storage. Did you know that two-thirds of the glycogen (the body's stored energy) is stockpiled in your muscle tissue? The more lean muscle you have, the more energy you have.

If you need still more motivation to start your weight-training program, keep in mind that less fat—and thus more muscle—means fewer wrinkles! According to research conducted at the University of Pennsylvania School of Medicine, people who exercise regularly have more resistance to wrinkles than those who don't. Increased blood supply to the skin means that more nutrients are keeping the skin healthy and glowing, while exercise helps to reduce the amount of fat under the skin. The closer the muscle is to the skin, the better the blood supply to the skin. Another study, directed by Dr. James White at the exercise physiology department at the University of California at San Diego, showed that in a group of sedentary middle-aged women the bags under their eyes disappeared only weeks after they began exercising. Talk about all-over results!

In the next chapter we'll show you how we designed programs to suit the bodies and needs of each of our models. They're women just like you, busy, active people; some are mothers, some are career-oriented, some active in sports, and not one of them ever dreamed she'd be lifting weights to reshape her body and her life. After you see and read about how it worked for them, we'll show you how to develop your own weight-training program to achieve the same fantastic results.

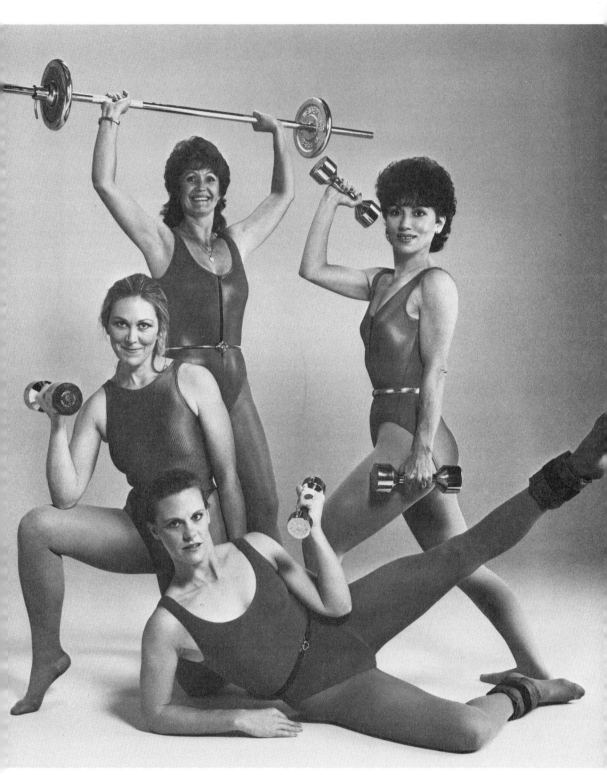

2

THE REAL BODY MAKEOVERS

JILL RICHARDSON

Age: 32	
Height: 5'3"	
Weight Before Program: 134	
Weight After Program: 118	

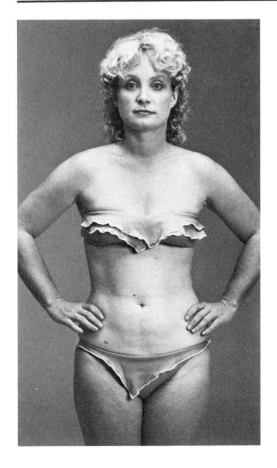 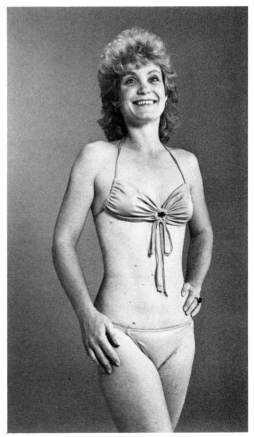

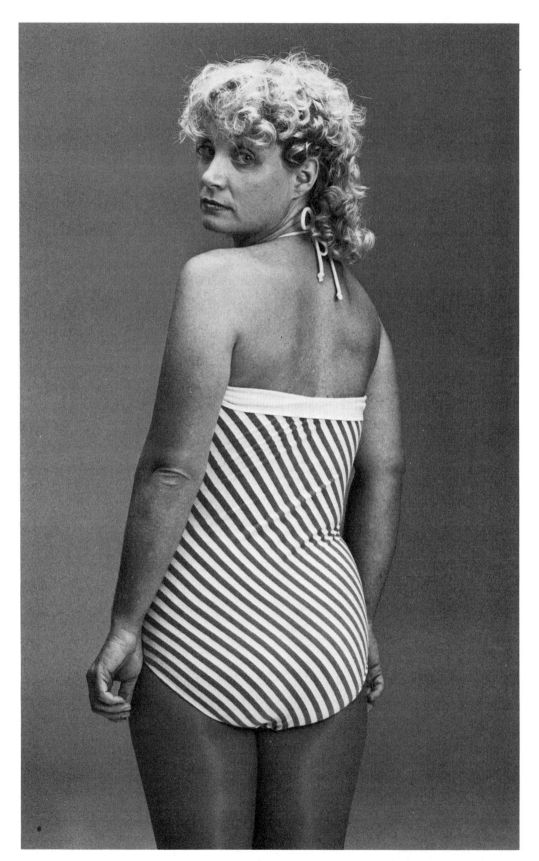

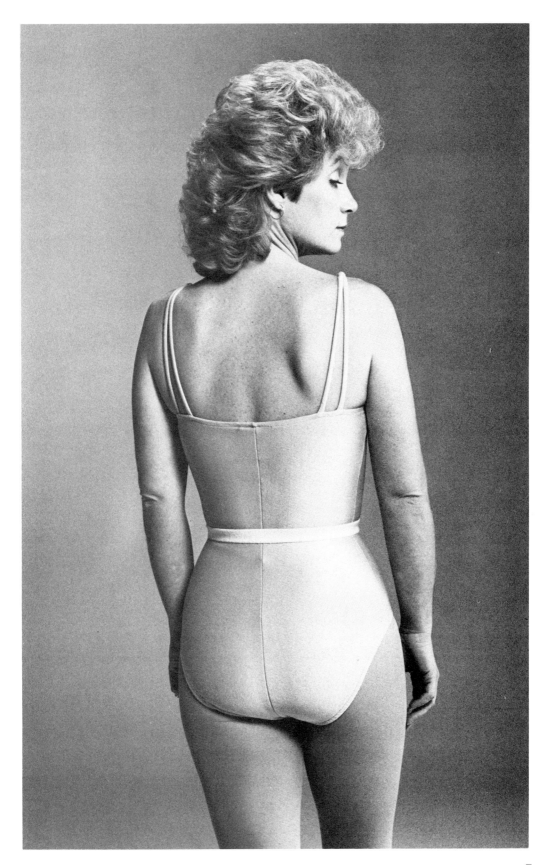

I always looked presentable in clothes; I don't think anyone would have called me "fat." But when I saw myself in the mirror just before taking a shower, I'd shudder. I *felt* fat, and that's what mattered. I didn't like the roll around my waist, my thighs weren't firm, and I just generally looked out of shape. I was far from the body I wanted to have.

When my lover and I broke up, I decided to go for the kind of body I wanted. I knew I could get it. Finding a new romance in my life was just the motivation I needed.

I had tried weight training before, but I'd injured myself. I wasn't using the proper grip, I was lifting weights that were too heavy, and I was doing a number of exercises that were unnecessary. I was also starting to look bulky instead of sleek. Now I realize that using the wrong exercises and weights that were too heavy was absolutely counterproductive!

After talking to Anita and Franco, I knew that with the right program I could be successful. For me, the "right program" meant doing all the exercises Franco and Anita suggested (except the squats and the bench press—I gave up on those) and constantly reminding myself of the body I wanted by using the visualization technique Anita taught me. I went through magazine after magazine looking for pictures of the kind of body I'd like to have. Finding the pictures wasn't as easy as it sounds. There are plenty of beautiful models in fashion magazines, but only a few of them really have the kind of body I want—or that I can realistically achieve. I'm not built long and lean, I'm short and curvaceous. I have a very feminine body that I had never learned to appreciate—I had always wanted to look like somebody else. My visualizations helped me learn that *my body* is wonderful. The weight-training program showed me how to redesign it to look its very best. Positive thinking helped enormously. So did giving away all my "fat" clothes. When I did that, I had no choice but to succeed.

Now I train 3 times a week, in the morning before going to work. As a television producer, my life is busy, so I still find it difficult to exercise 4 times a week, which is my new goal. If I miss even 1 session, I feel bloated, sluggish, and irritable.

I'd say that I'm three-quarters of the way to the body I want to have. I still have some trouble spots—my stomach and my rear end need firming. But just arriving at the point where I finally can say that I *like* my body is a major accomplishment.

The positive reinforcement I've received from people around me has been wonderful. Everybody—honestly *everybody*—comments on how fantastic I look. Now I can wear clothes I like, and feel happier and more attractive. Weight training has made a difference in my life. I'm determined to stick with it.

There have been other big plusses: I completely gave up smoking (why punish a great new body?), and there's a new, wonderful man in my life. When I said weight training made a difference, I meant it!

OUR ANALYSIS OF JILL'S BODY

Jill is an endomorph: She's naturally curvy. Slim ankles and wrists, slim calves, and a bit too much padding everywhere else. With one look, we knew that Jill had the potential for a gorgeous body: narrow waist, firm bust line, narrow hips, and slim thighs. She just had to burn off the fat that was hiding all of her body's assets. See how completely it responded: Her shoulders widened slightly, her midriff tightened, and her waist slimmed by a full 3 inches, as did her hips. Her stomach flattened, and she lost a total of 5½ inches from her thighs.

Jill started on the basic program, doing 25 repetitions of each exercise with no breaks between sets, and no weights. This rapid motion helped burn fat, and that was our initial goal. Then, as she got stronger, we added more reps and 5-pound dumbbells to help define her muscles. To trim her abdomen she did a full set of stomach exercises every day, and added lunges to slim her thighs. The lunges added a firm, round curve to her rear end. Her new, more erect posture also helps give a long, lean line to her body, accenting her trimmer proportions.

Jill's determination made a big difference in the way she progressed. She is a very positive thinker who knows how to set and achieve goals. It was no surprise that she accomplished what she set out to do: She was mentally and physically prepared for the challenge of redesigning her body.

JILL'S RESULTS:

	BEFORE	AFTER	INCHES LOST
Upper Arms	11½"	10"	3 (1½" each)
Forearms	9¼"	9"	½" (each ¼")
Bust	34"	32½"	1½"
Waist	27"	24"	3"
Abdomen	34¾"	30"	4¾"
Hips	38"	35"	3"
Thighs	22¾"	20"	5½" (2¾" each)
Calves	14¼"	13¼"	2" (each 1")

Total Inches Lost: 23½"
Total Weight Lost: 16 pounds

ALISON ELDER

Age: 29

Height: 5'3"

Weight Before Program: 126¼

Weight After Program: 119

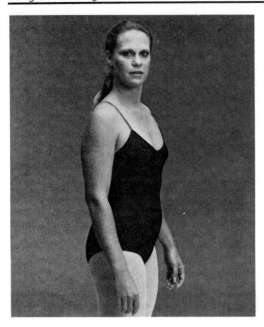 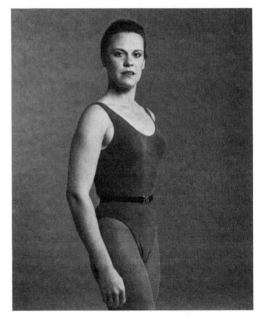

I am now at an age where losing weight is becoming increasingly difficult. As an accountant, I sit at a desk for 8 hours a day, so I was afraid that before long I would look fat and middle-aged, with a broad, flabby rear-view. I didn't want to get hopelessly out of shape.

Although I never followed a regular daily workout routine, I've always been an active person. Before I injured my knee skiing, I always skiied 3 days a week in the winter, and hiked and windsurfed in the summer. I tried aerobics classes and swimming, too, but I never really saw big changes in my body. I went on crash diets intermittently and always lost weight, but the weight loss didn't last. I wanted a noticeable, permanent change—and I wanted it quickly.

As soon as I started the Columbus' weight-training program, I saw immediate changes which motivated me further. My jeans became loose in the waist and hips after just 2 weeks of working out. After just 1 month of weight training, I bought new ones, a full size smaller. I was amazed. Now I am constantly getting compliments from my friends and family. I feel I really look good.

There were times when I didn't want to do the calf exercises or the wide-grip pull-downs. They were hard. But I kept after myself. I kept in mind that failing to do an exercise would mean slowing down my progress. I'd only be hurting myself. So I very rarely skipped any exercises.

I suppose the biggest thrill of all is knowing that I can stick with something that's good for me. I've never done that before; I didn't think I ever could adhere to an exercise routine. I learned a lesson: The things that are the easiest to continue are those that show results, make me feel good, and don't make me crazy.

Now I enjoy my workouts. I exercise 3 days a week with weights and go to an aerobics class 3 times a week. I found that I do my best weight training after work at about 7:00 (I work out for about 45 minutes). I fit the aerobics in whenever I can, either before or after work.

When I first started the program, it was important to me to slim my thighs, tone my arms, flatten my stomach, and lose at least 15 pounds. My thighs have slimmed by about 2 inches. Thanks to the triceps exercise, my arms are no longer flabby in back, and the crunches have strengthened my abdominals. After I gave up eating dairy products and stuck with a low-calorie, low-fat nutritional program, I was disappointed at first that I didn't lose more weight. Now I realize that even though I don't look muscular, my body weight has shifted from fat to lean weight. I guess it's true that muscle weighs more than fat.

I'm really happy, and I'm not the least bit ashamed of my body anymore. I have to admit, I look as good as I feel.

OUR ANALYSIS OF ALISON'S BODY

Alison is naturally thin, an ectomorph. Her problem was that she had slowly gained a few extra pounds that had added width at her waist, a few too many inches around her abdomen and hips, and pockets of extra fat on her thighs. Her problems weren't serious, but she was out of proportion for her lean build. Her shoulders needed to be developed somewhat, her waist needed to be trimmed, and her hips and thighs needed firming. She had great potential—and a lot of drive, which always helps.

Like so many ectomorphs, she didn't need to lose a great deal of fat. Her body simply needed to develop more muscle. The energy used to build her lean body mass would easily burn off any excess fat.

Notice that Alison lost only 7¼ pounds, yet her total inch loss was 18½ inches, including more than 4 inches off her abdomen and 2 inches off each thigh. The inch loss proves what weight trainers have always known: muscle is heavier and denser than fat. Therefore, a newly reshaped thigh with more lean body mass instead of flabby fat will be considerably thinner than it was before, yet it may weigh exactly the same. In Alison's case, we estimate that she lost about 12¼ pounds of fat—and gained 5 pounds of new lean tissue. Her net loss was 7¼ pounds *and* all those inches.

For women with ectomorphic bodies like Alison's, it's imperative to use heavy weights and fewer reps. While endomorphic Jill might have done 3 sets of 35 lunges with 5-pound dumbbells to trim her thighs, Alison did 3 sets of 15 lunges using a 20- or 30-pound barbell. They both achieved the same slim results, but each had to do it her own way.

ALISON'S RESULTS

	BEFORE	AFTER	INCHES LOST
Upper Arms	11½"	10½"	2" (1" each)
Forearms	9½"	9"	1" (½" each)
Bust	34¾"	34"	¾"
Waist	29"	25½"	3½"
Abdomen	34¼"	29¾"	4½"
Hips	36¾"	34½"	2¼"
Thighs	22¾"	20¾"	4" (2" each)
Calves	12½"	12¼"	½" (¼" each)

Total Inches Lost: 18½"
Total Weight Lost: 7¼ pounds

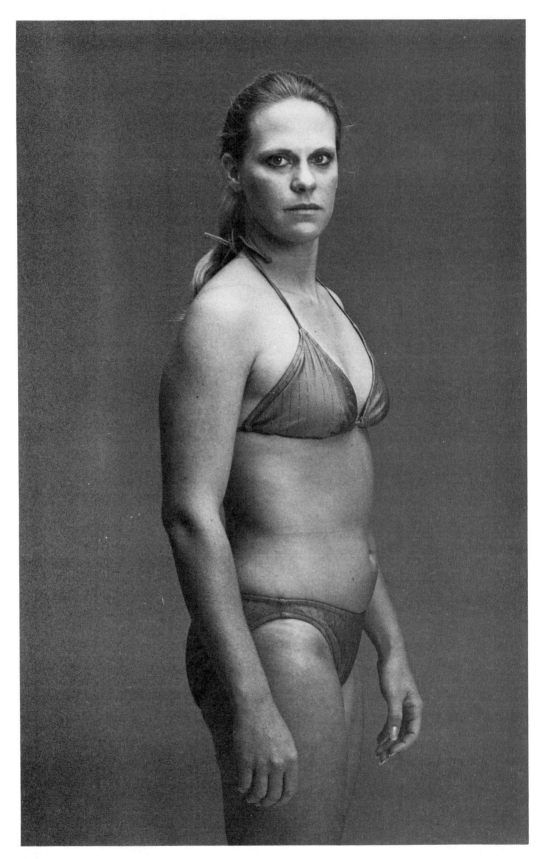

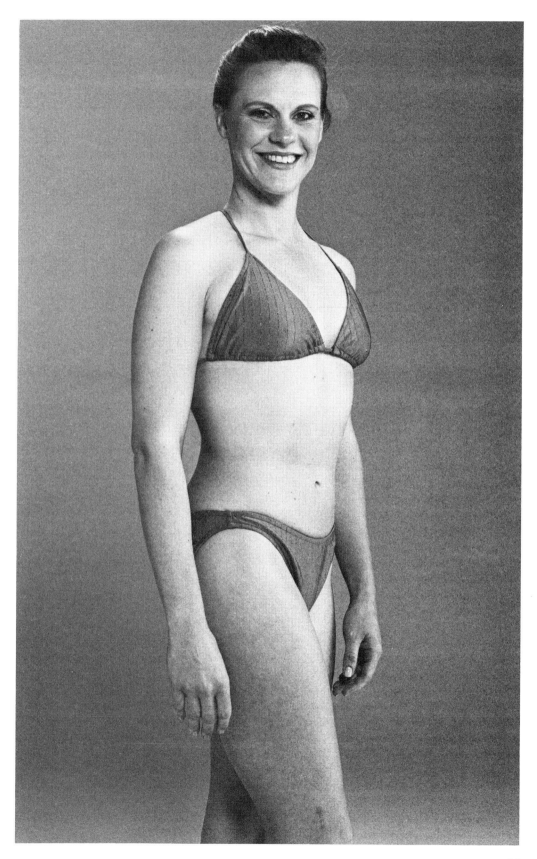

GINI GRUBER

Age: 51

Height: 5'5"

Weight Before Program: 154½

Weight After Program: 133½

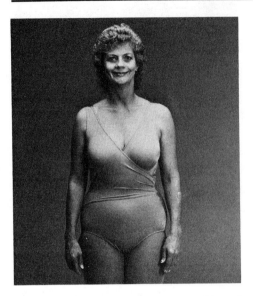 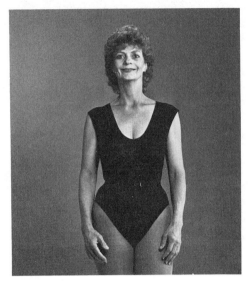

As the executive vice-president of a food-allergies testing laboratory, I felt it was important to look fit and healthy instead of flabby. When I started this weight-training program I knew my eating patterns were out of control. That was not consistent with the basic tenets of my career, nor with my own personality; I'm basically a disciplined person. And I knew, too, that I wasn't getting any younger. It was time to do something to help myself.

When I tipped the scale at 154, I almost cried. I hadn't been this heavy since I was pregnant. My kids are now 26, 24, 22, and 20—I couldn't use pregnancy weight gain as an excuse! Frankly, there were no excuses left. I made the commitment both to myself and to the Columbus. I was determined to succeed.

In the past I had tried every kind of reducing plan. I had no success with Weight Watchers. I lost a lot on Dr. Atkins's diet, but it didn't stay off. And the last time I tried it, I didn't lose any weight—I'd lose and then immediately gain the weight back. Believe me, I am a diet expert. I know the whys and wherefore of all the different regimes. What I needed was a *sensible* food program. I had blood tests done to determine my food allergies; these are called cytotoxic tests. I found that I am highly allergic to wheat, yeast, coffee, and lettuce. So when Franco and Anita suggested that I cut out sugar and dairy products, reduce the other fats in my diet and cut way down on complex carbohydrate intake, it made sense to me. I tried to eliminate dairy products, red meat, and bread. That was it. My calories were not cut drastically; I'd say I consume about 1,200 calories each day. In 90 days I lost 21 pounds.

The weight training made all the difference. Six days a week I got up at 5:00 A.M. and exercised for 2 hours. I missed my workouts only about 3 times in 3 months. I'm proud to say I was—and still am—extremely dedicated to doing something good for *me*. I don't always like working out, but I enjoy the mental and physical high I feel after the training sessions.

Leg exercises give me the most trouble, but I never skip them, grueling as they may be. I tell myself that if I want thin legs, I have to do the leg raises, the back hip lifts, and the squats.

14

I started to see results in 3 weeks. That was great motivation. Now I can wear clothes I haven't been able to wear for years. And I can see my pelvic bones, which had been buried for years!

I like the way I look so much better now. I haven't yet achieved everything I want. My thighs could be firmer, and my stomach should be flatter. But I'm convinced that I can accomplish this too. Everything I've achieved so far was done with free weights. And now I am ready to incorporate some outdoor exercises into my program too. Maybe I'll try walking or tennis, or swimming as the weather gets warmer.

I'm also pleased that I have finally begun to integrate new eating habits into my daily life. I don't feel the need to clean my plate anymore—I stop when I'm full. I've regained control of my eating. I still have an occasional eating binge, usually triggered by emotional stress, but I'm aware when those times are coming and can usually keep the binge within limits.

My family has been very supportive of my efforts. My husband loves my new body—in fact, it's inspired him to see the Columbus about a weight-training program for himself!

OUR ANALYSIS OF GINI'S BODY

Gini's body presented all the problems of a typical overweight endomorph. She had more fat than muscle so she was plump all over, with extra bulk below the waist, especially at her stomach, hips, and thighs. Like many women of her age, her upper arms were flabby and needed work in the triceps region.

The major thrust of Gini's program was to burn fat, to eliminate the thick blanket of fat that concealed her natural form. By doing plenty of fast repetitions, with almost no breaks between sets, she literally watched the fat melt away. In 2 weeks she had lost more than 5 inches—2¾ inches from her abdomen alone! Endomorphs see the fastest results because spot-reducing builds muscle and burns fat in very specific places. Since muscle is so much denser than fat, flabby areas respond quickly. Although we gave her no specific exercises to decrease her bust line, her bust measurement showed a 2¾-inch loss, which resulted in a firmer, more youthful silhouette. One-arm rowing exercises strengthened her upper back and improved her posture, and in so doing lifted her breasts about 2 inches.

Gini used light weights—never more than 5-pound dumbbells and 5-pound ankle weights, but she did 50 repetitions of many of the exercises. Her total weight loss was 21 pounds, and she lost 28¾ inches in 90 days.

GINI'S RESULTS

	BEFORE	AFTER	INCHES LOST
Upper Arms	11¼"	10¼"	2" (1" each)
Forearms	9¼"	8¼"	2" (1" each)
Bust	38¼"	35½"	2¾"
Waist	29"	25½"	3½"
Abdomen	39"	33"	6"
Hips	40½"	37"	3½"
Thighs	24½"	21¾"	5½" (2¾" each)
Calves	14½"	12¾"	3½" (1¾" each)

Total Inches Lost: 28¾"
Total Weight Lost: 21 pounds

15

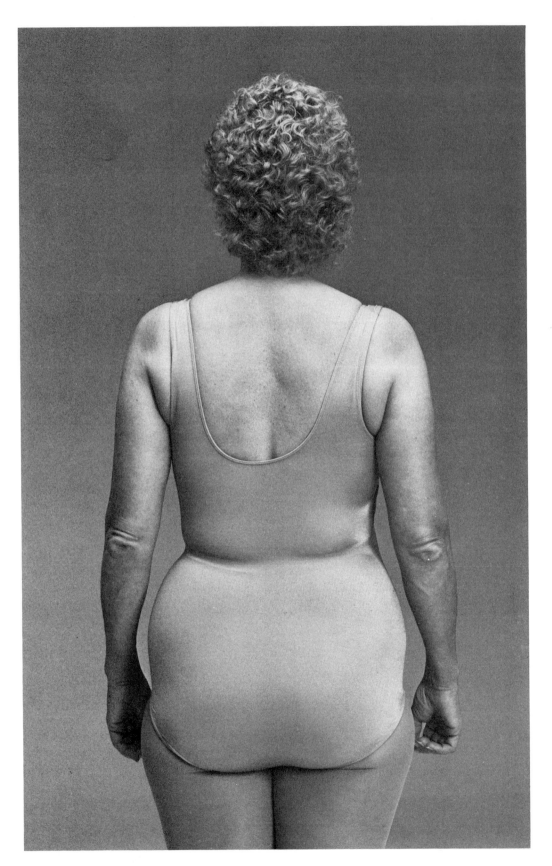

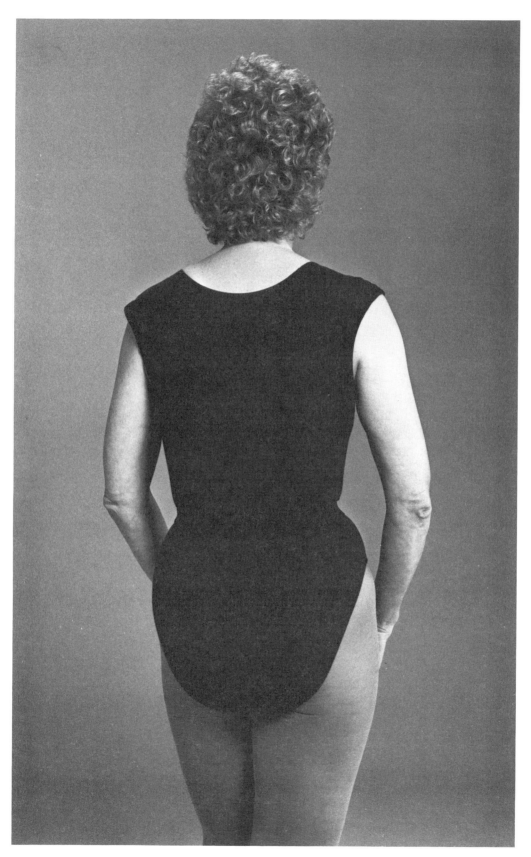

ELEANOR SOBEL

Age:	33
Height:	5'2"
Weight Before Program:	94
Weight After Program:	97

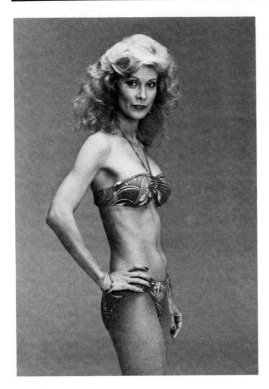
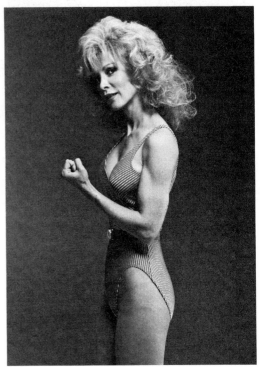

I was thin all my life, and hated it. I never wore sleeveless clothes because I felt self-conscious about my skinny arms. I never felt very sexy. When I mentally pictured myself, I envisioned a slim person, but the mirror always reflected the truth: *skinny*.

I had tried any number of ways to gain weight. I ate constantly, but couldn't gain. There were times when I'd envy average or overweight people—at least they could skip a meal if they wanted to. If I skip a meal, I lose weight.

So when Franco and Anita said they could help me build up my body, I was ready to try. The first thing I did was to find a picture of the body I wanted mine to look like. I chose a photo of Candy Csencsits, one of the champion body builders. She's petite like me, but she has incredible definition. She has curves in all the right places, but she doesn't look like a guy, bulging with muscles. So I kept that mental image: Candy's body with my head on it!

Then I started working out, and eating more protein and complex carbohydrates. I worked out every day for 1½ to 2 hours. I'm a cosmetologist and electrologist, so my day starts early and ends late. Some nights I don't get home until 8:00. Then by the time I cook dinner for my husband and me and play with the dogs for a few minutes, it's 9:30 or 10:00 before I start working out. But I'm diligent. If I skip a session, I feel like I'm cheating my body.

The lower body exercises were the hardest for me. Sometimes I had to talk to my legs and say "harder, stronger," and "you can do it"—just to encourage them to go on, to get one more push out of them. But look, it works! My legs look better. The flabby part of my thighs became firm curves, and my calves are actually shapely. My arms look wonderful. In 90 days they each increased by ¾ inch. I'm eager to see what happens in 6 months.

I love to work out now. It gives me great pleasure to see the results I've achieved. And the people who teased me when I told them I was lifting weights have had to eat their words. The changes are obvious; my new shape is *very* attractive. Now instead of getting ribbed, I'm getting complimented!

The best part of all this is that I *love* my body now. I can wear sexy clothes and feel good about myself in them. For a treat, I just went out and bought two ultra-sexy bikinis. What a great feeling!

OUR ANALYSIS OF ELEANOR'S BODY

Eleanor had the kind of body some women consider ideal. But to our trained eyes, she was too thin, with no muscle definition and pockets of fat on her thighs and buttocks. It may be hard for you to believe that a 94-pound woman has fat to lose, but look at Eleanor's "before" photos. Notice her thighs and rear end. Those were bulges on an otherwise too-thin body. We call her problem "skinny-fat."

Like Alison, Eleanor is an ectomorph, but unlike Alison, she had almost no developed muscles—no feminine curves to shape her lean silhouette. She also lacked strength and stamina. She couldn't start out with a program of heavy weights—the kind that builds muscles—because she couldn't lift the weights. She had to build up strength and develop endurance.

We taught her to do limited, slow repetitions (about half as many as endomorphs do—12 to 15) with progressively heavier weights. We also instructed Eleanor to increase her protein intake substantially, while keeping fats to a minimum. This additional protein helped build new lean body mass.

Following this routine, her body quickly developed curves, and the saddlebags disappeared just as rapidly. Because she didn't have much fat to work off, it was easier for Eleanor to concentrate on building up her problem areas: her upper arms, her shoulders, and her back.

Her weight gain reflects the muscles and strength she developed, yet her figure is extremely feminine and beautiful. Notice that overall she lost only ½ inch, but if you look at each specific change in her figure, she gained in all the right spots and lost inches exactly where she wanted to. Now her waist is even tinier, making her enhanced bust line look even larger. Her hips and thighs have slimmed to gorgeous curves, and her shoulders and arms have a lean but shapely definition.

ELEANOR'S RESULTS

	BEFORE	AFTER	INCHES LOST
Upper Arms	8¼"	9"	1½" (¾" each) (GAINED)
Forearms	7½"	7½"	0
Bust	31"	32½"	1½" (GAINED)
Waist	23½"	22"	1½"
Abdomen	28½"	27"	1½"
Hips	32½"	33"	½" (GAINED)
Thighs	18¾"	18¼"	1" (½" each)
Calves	12"	12"	0"

Total Inches Lost: ½"
Total Weight Gain: 3 pounds

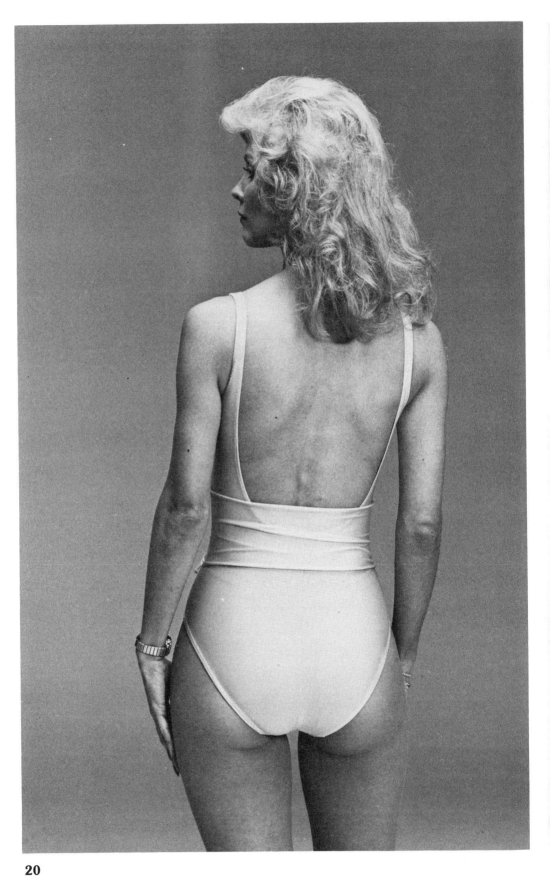

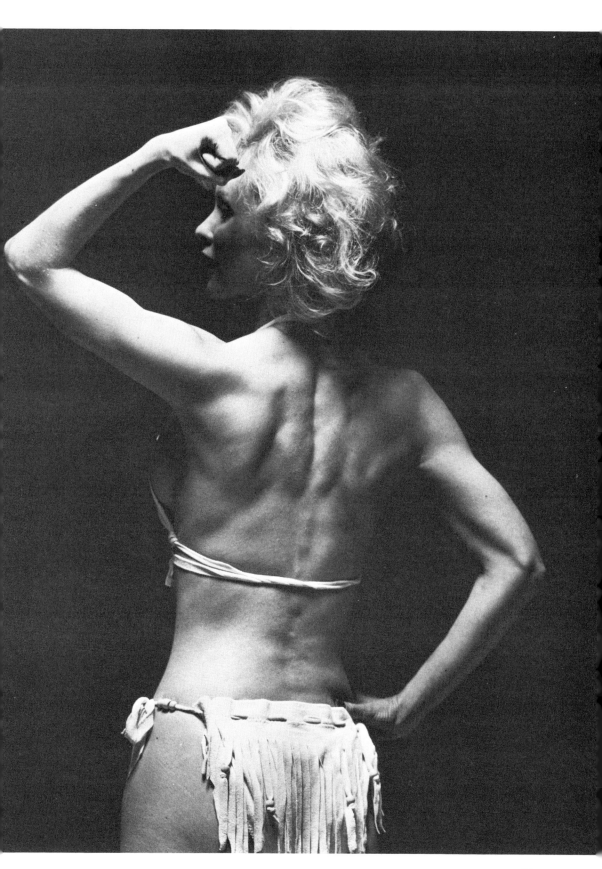

DR. ALYSE DANIEL

Age: 35	
Height: 5'3"	
Weight before program: 143	
Weight After Program: 131	

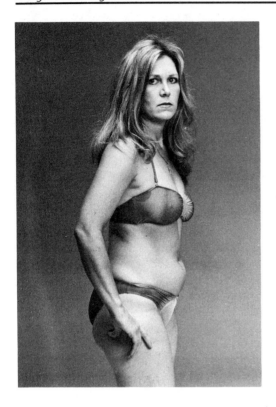 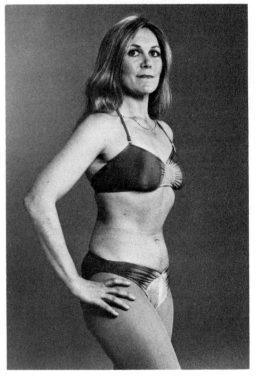

Exercise means more to me than just getting my body in shape. In so many ways it's a reflection of how I'm getting my life in shape too. You see, I've wanted to improve my total self-image for a long time.

I've tried many different methods with only temporary success. But now I finally have the willingness and incentive to succeed.

I try to exercise with free weights every day for at least 20 minutes. I do stomach work, leg lifts, lunges, squats, stretches, and waist exercises 5 to 7 times a week. I have no set time for my workouts. I find that I train just as well in the morning as in the afternoon or evening, so I fit it into my schedule whenever possible. Since I am a chiropractor and a musician, I have a very busy schedule, but I've made my training periods a top priority.

I started seeing results almost immediately. Weight started to drop off consistently, but when I reached a point I couldn't get past, I realized I was eating compulsively. I had to face that fact and decide exactly what my priorities were. I started exercising more and eating a little less, and I totally eliminated dairy products. Now, the more I work out, the more positive benefits I receive; my new eating habits enhance the results.

My thighs, waist, and buttocks still need work, but I look and feel so much better. My physical image is closer to what I want it to be. Like the work of art a sculptor shapes, the changes in my body have been gradual but important.

Positive feedback is secondary to me, although many people have paid me compliments about my body. What really matters is how I feel about myself. And I'm feeling much better. Weight training will continue to be a part of my life.

22

OUR ANALYSIS OF ALYSE'S BODY

A body like Alyse's poses a challenge. She is a mesomorph, a balanced structure with a potential for lean muscle mass, but she has a great deal of solid fat distributed evenly over her body. She's not flabby—in fact, her fat is so solid it could be mistaken for muscle. Some mesomorphs carry their weight that way, and it's difficult to break down the fat.

She needed to exchange her adipose tissue for lean body mass. So first, her program had to help her body burn calories fast, using up as much of her stored fat as possible. Then we had to change the program so that she could define her curves by developing her natural musculature.

We suggested that she follow our basic training program, but we increased her reps very quickly. After 2 weeks she was doing 40 reps of each exercise, and in 2 more weeks she was up to 50 reps. When she started using weights, she used light, 5-pound weights and continued the high reps. With every session she worked up a sweat and burned calories very quickly. Her body responded immediately.

During her sixth week, Alyse's weight increased by more than 1 pound, so we analyzed her diet. She admitted that she had been eating compulsively. Talking about it helped; she got back on track and showed a 5-pound loss in the next 2 weeks. She also increased her training program during that time, so she burned even more calories.

As you can see from her before-and-after pictures, Alyse's results are remarkable. She lost a total of 20½ inches, including 4 inches from her waist and more than 5 from her abdomen. During the last 2 weeks of her training program, she nipped a full 2 inches from her waist by increasing her lying side leg lifts to 3 sets of 50 reps each.

At this point Alyse is concentrating on thigh- and buttocks-firming exercises, both areas that will respond quickly now that she has learned to control her eating and increase her level of exercise.

ALYSE'S RESULTS

	BEFORE	AFTER	INCHES LOST
Upper Arms	11¼"	10½"	1½" (¾" each)
Forearms	9"	8¾"	½" (¼" each)
Bust	35¾"	33½"	2¼"
Waist	30"	26"	4"
Abdomen	35¼"	30"	5¼"
Hips	39½"	37"	2½"
Thighs	23"	21"	4" (2" each)
Calves	14¼"	14"	¼" (total ½")

Total Inches Lost: 20½"
Total Weight Lost: 12 pounds

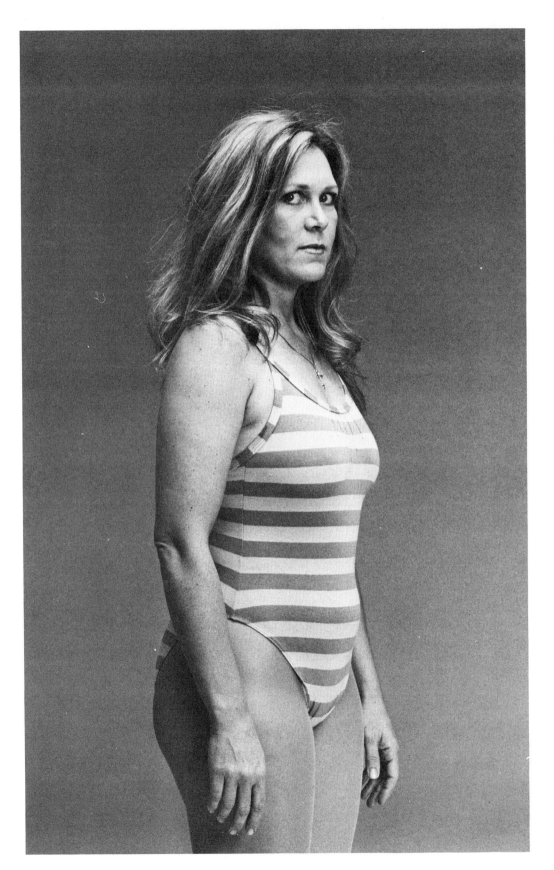

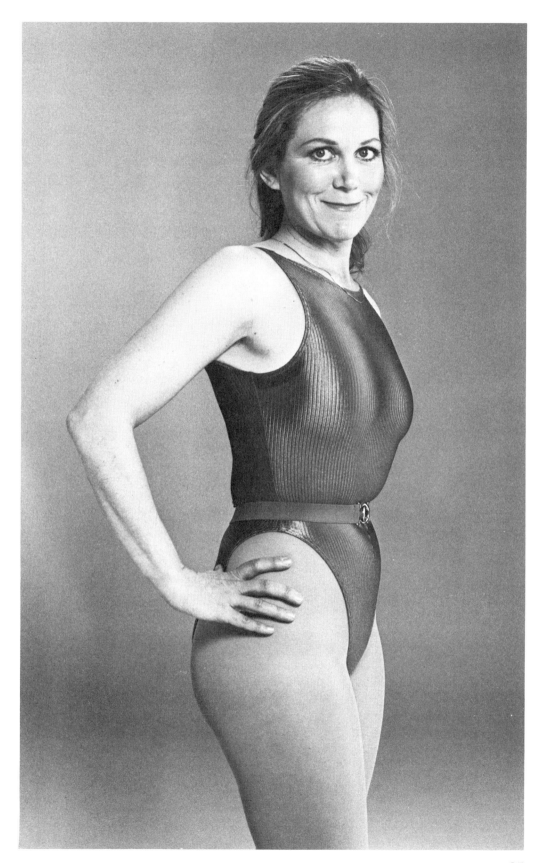

SUZETTE L. SMITH

Age: 38	
Height: 5'3½"	
Weight Before Program: 138	
Weight After Program: 129	

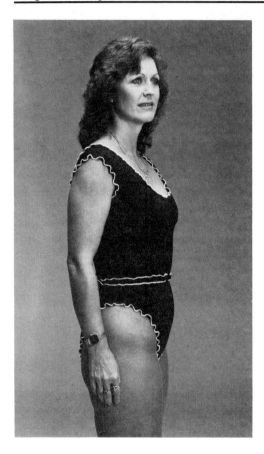 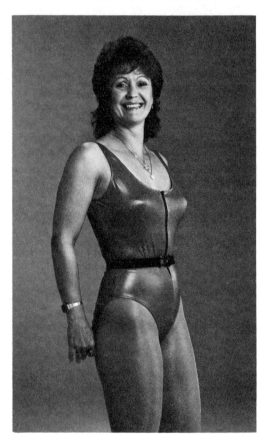

It's not going to sound very dramatic when I tell you that I lost 9 pounds. That's my progress in the last 90 days. But you should have seen me 6 months ago! That's when 162 pounds of fat hung on my 5' 3½" frame. I looked awful, I felt awful about myself, and I felt as if I were a hopeless case.

I was lucky that I discovered weight training then; it saved me. Maybe that sounds a bit evangelistic, but that's how I feel. You must understand that I had spent all of my adult life battling fat. There I was, nearing the ripe old age of 38, and I looked 15 years older and moved as though I were 20 years older. I was an ugly mess. I wanted to achieve body mastery while I was still young enough to enjoy it, and while my body was still young enough to respond to the program I chose.

By the time I started this program with Franco and Anita, I was desperate. With their guidance, I lost 24 pounds and discovered my waist, my hip bones, and my knees. No part of me was hidden any longer with fat. But I was still a bit scared. I had lost hundreds of pounds in my lifetime, and I had always gained them back. I was determined to win this time. After 3 months Franco revised my program to improve my body: tighten my buttocks, flatten my tummy, and firm my thighs. After I actually started to see those things happen, I was hooked on fitness. I wanted to hone my body—to get it in the best possible shape. I didn't want to face 40 with any regrets about my body. And I won't.

For the last 6 months I have consistently trained for 30 to 45 minutes, 5 days a week, and I go to an aerobics class for 1 hour 5 days a week. I play tennis twice a week. That's a lot of exercise, but I love it. I know that exercise can help me to achieve all the goals I want for my body, as well as making me feel energized all the time. Weight training has become a way of life for me now, and I can't imagine wanting to stop. I feel and look so much better. I am in charge of my body, and *I* can determine how it looks. That's been an extremely important realization.

It hasn't all been easy. Some of the exercises are hard to do. But they work. The leg exercises were the ones I resisted the most, especially the lunges and squats. However, after doing them consistently for one month, I lost 4 inches off my thighs—and promptly decided to love them.

My entire body looks like a sculpture now. My arms, chest, back, waist, and legs all have definition. When I was a teenager I weighed less than I do now, but even then my middle still looked like a sauage. Now I feel like a million, and look like a million. When I run into old friends who haven't seen me in a year, they can't believe it. They all want to know the secret of my success. And of course, I tell them it's weight training. I want everyone to feel as good about themselves as I do.

OUR ANALYSIS OF SUZETTE'S BODY

Suzette has worked with us for 6 months—although the "before" pictures you see here were taken after 3 months of work. She was much heavier when she began, as you see in the inset photo taken when she was at her heaviest, a few months before she started weight training. During the time that the other women in this chapter were following beginner and intermediate programs, Suzette followed an advanced program geared for professional body builders. Her new goal is to enter a body-building competition.

When we first met Suzette she was carrying around 162 pounds on a petite frame. And most of the fat was below her waist. Her body was both misshapen and unhealthy. Even under all that extra fat, however, we could tell that Suzette was a mesomorph with exceptional potential for developing a beautiful body. Her body was meant to be lean and fabulous, with gently defined muscles adding feminine curves. We told her it was very possible to have the kind of body she had always dreamed about. We also told her that it would take time, but the results would be worth it. We weren't sure she was convinced that she *could* attain her dream body, but we were underestimating the strength of her positive attitude. She was hooked on fitness in no time and ready to pursue a training program that only the most dedicated weight trainers undertake.

But she started out just like everyone else. She had to fit her program into her busy life as a wife, mother, and professional goal-setting consultant. She got organized, established her priorities, and found time in her day for everything that she wanted to do.

Her initial program consisted of a typical highly aerobic fat-burning routine of many quick reps—the same program we would assign to overweight endomorphs. But as she began to shed the weight and excess fat, it became clear that her muscles were ready for action. And so was she. In less than 3 months Suzette had made dramatic changes in her body. She was in control. She constantly readjusted her goals as she saw exactly how far her program allowed her to take charge of her body.

After her first 3 months' work she had lost 4 inches from her bust, 3 inches from her waist, 6 inches from her hips, 2½ inches from her abdomen, and 3 inches from her thighs. Though she was delighted with those results, she demanded still more of herself and asked for an advanced program. She was ready to sculpt her body into perfect proportions. Look at those results! Great proportions, and major losses right where she wanted them. She trimmed another 2½ inches from her waist, 1½ inches from her tummy, 3 more inches from her hips

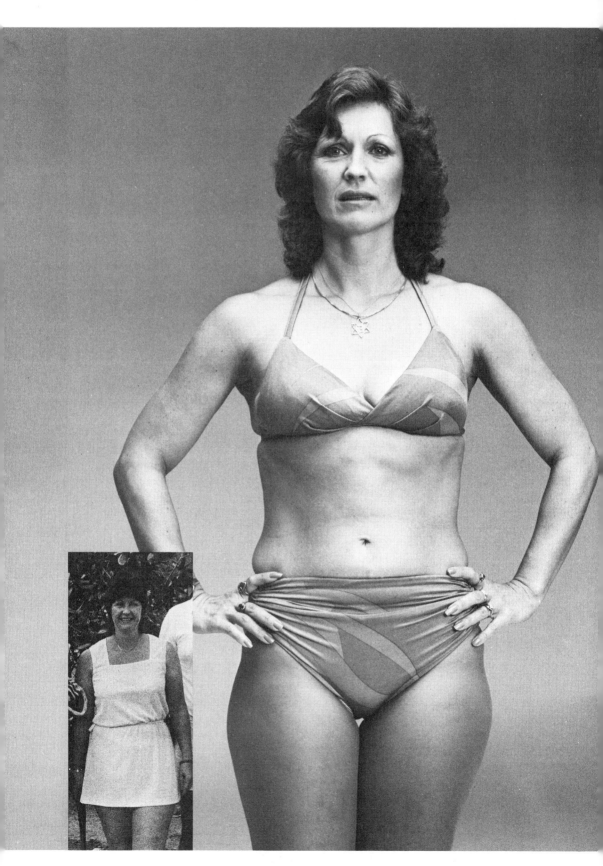

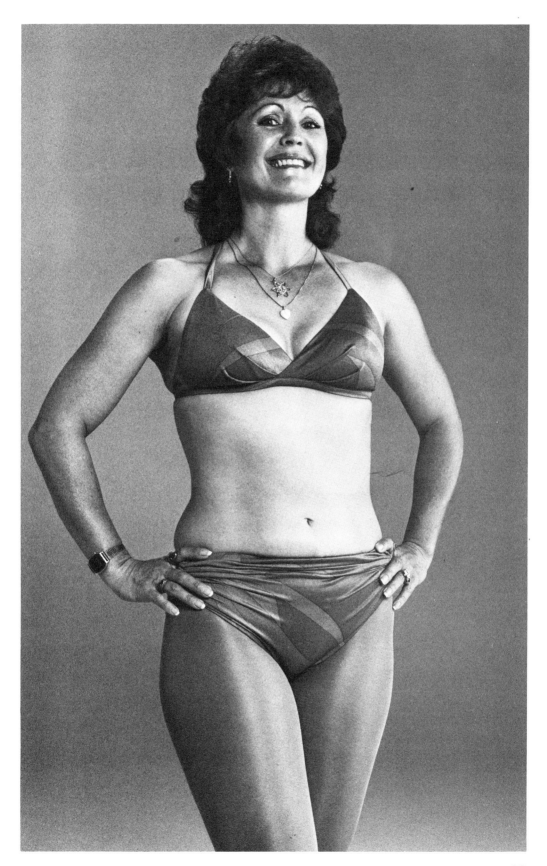

and a phenomenal total of 5 more inches from her thighs. We predict that in another 6 months Suzette will be ready for her first competition. She will work to define her back muscles, tighten her midriff and abdomen, and firm her thighs even more. But when it comes to a noncompetition body, Suzette has already achieved a winning silhouette.

SUZETTE'S RESULTS

	BEFORE	AFTER 90 DAYS	AFTER 180 DAYS	INCHES LOST
Upper Arms	11"	10½"	10¼"	1½" (¾" each)
Forearms	9½"	9"	8¾"	1½" (¾" each)
Bust	40"	36"	35½"	4½"
Waist	31"	28"	25½"	5½"
Abdomen	36"	33½"	31"	5"
Hips	43"	37"	34"	9"
Thighs	26"	24"	21½"	9" (4½" each)
Calves	15"	14½"	14½"	1" (½" each)

Total Inches Lost (90 days): **22"**
Total Inches Lost (180 days): **36"**
Total Weight Lost (90 days): **9 pounds**
Total Weight Lost (180 days): **41 pounds**

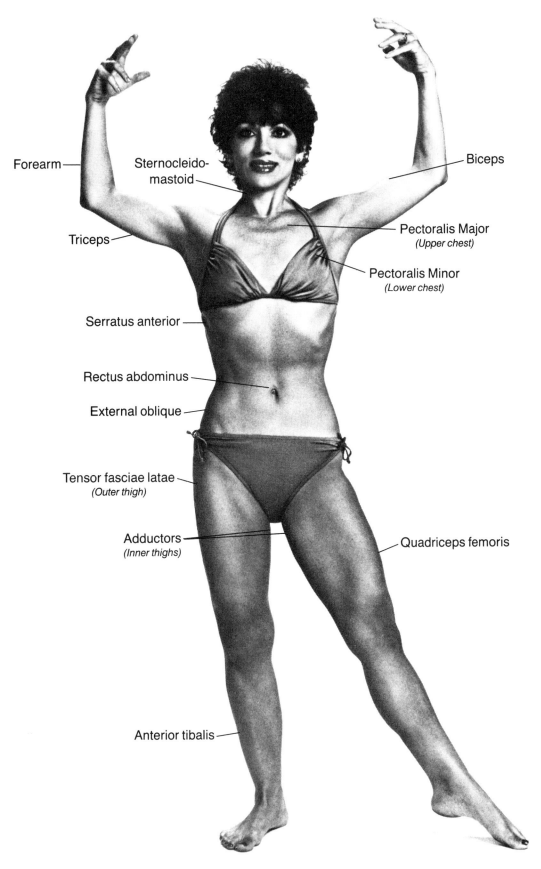

Forearm —

Sternocleido-
mastoid —

Triceps —

Serratus anterior —

Rectus abdominus —

External oblique —

Tensor fasciae latae —
(Outer thigh)

Adductors —
(Inner thighs)

Anterior tibalis —

Biceps

Pectoralis Major
(Upper chest)

Pectoralis Minor
(Lower chest)

Quadriceps femoris

31

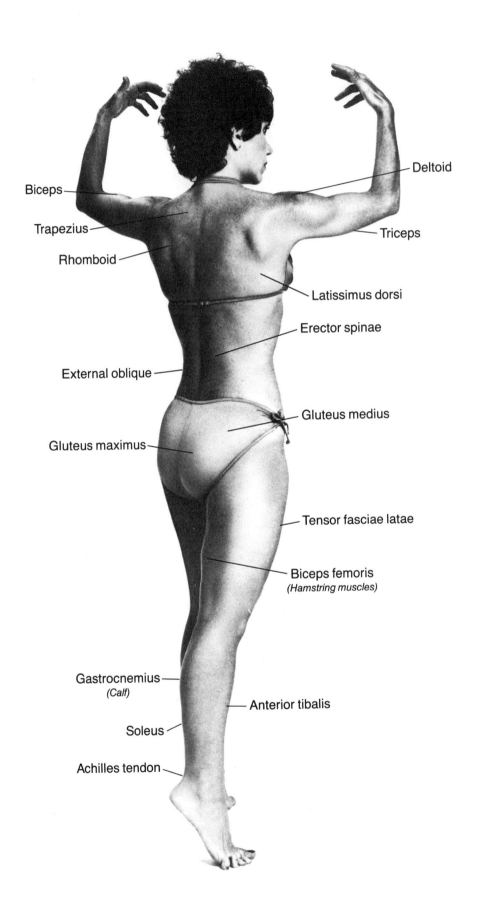

Deltoid

Biceps

Trapezius

Triceps

Rhomboid

Latissimus dorsi

Erector spinae

External oblique

Gluteus medius

Gluteus maximus

Tensor fasciae latae

Biceps femoris
(Hamstring muscles)

Gastrocnemius
(Calf)

Anterior tibalis

Soleus

Achilles tendon

3

SETTING YOUR GOALS

There's no such thing as a perfect body. Your goal should not be an impossible-to-achieve perfection, but simply a trimmer, healthier body—one that you enjoy and are proud of. A too-thin body is unattractive and unhealthy. A slim, firm, athletic body is not only good-looking, it is vital and filled with energy.

The women you just met in Chapter 2 have learned a very important lesson. They no longer think of nutrition in terms of crash diets they can climb on or fall off as the mood hits them. They no longer see exercise as an activity to be confined to sporadic weekend workouts. Both good nutrition and a balanced weight-training/exercise program have become integral parts of their daily lives. And, in allowing this to happen, they have left behind exaggerated swings in their weight, fitness, health, self-image, and self-confidence.

They have learned the lesson that we believe is most important: "The road to success is always under construction" (quoted recently in the *Hollywood Reporter*). They know that they can be flexible, because they have the knowledge and the awareness to determine for themselves what works for them.

In this book, we will offer you many choices of excellent weight-training programs, but ultimately it is you who will have to work out your own individual program. We can give you the information upon which to base your decisions. But we trust you to choose wisely, since you know your body best.

Remember: You are in control.

You are reading this book and following the programs we describe because you want to be shapelier, more attractive *and* happier *and* healthier. You will not achieve those goals through overtraining. Health, happiness, and attractiveness are the result of mind and body in harmony. You can achieve that harmony by learning how to be both disciplined *and* kind to yourself: disciplined in choosing a program and sticking with it; kind by recognizing and appreciating your attributes and forgiving your temporary setbacks. You are a thinking, feeling person, one with both strengths and weaknesses. Learn to accept and appreciate all the things that make you unique.

You've probably already wasted countless hours and dollars looking for quick results. There are no easy answers, and no overnight programs to give you good health and an attractive body. The only lasting improvement will come with consistency, balance, and a positive mental attitude. Combine these qualities with the programs we've designed for you in this book, and you will not only avoid overtraining, you will maintain your new body for as long as you want it. Forever, we hope.

POSITIVE THINKING EQUALS POSITIVE RESULTS

What adjectives would you use if someone asked you to describe yourself right now? Would you mentally cringe and allow words like "fat," "unattractive," or worse to creep into your mind? Or would you permit yourself to recognize all the beautiful things about yourself that make you special? Can you appreciate the uniquely talented person you are? Can you finally allow yourself to be all that you really want to be? If so, you have taken the most important step toward reaching your goals—whether they relate to weight, fitness, or any other part of your life. If you really think it, you can make it so.

You are going to start seeing yourself as you want to be—slim, healthy, active, attractive, and successful. Yes, successful, because that's what you'll be: successful in taking control of your life.

Remember, the past doesn't count. All that matters is the present and the future. Use the present to make your future the way you want it to be. Use your creative energies to visualize your body and your life as you want them to be.

Remember, too, that your attitude will determine your success. In his book *The Power of Positive Thinking*, Dr. Norman Vincent Peale lists four steps necessary to achieve success. We believe they are as relevant to redesigning your body as they are to other areas of your life.

First, you must decide exactly what it is you want. In terms of your body, this might translate into fitting into a pair of jeans you've always dreamed of wearing. Or perhaps there's a dress size you've been wanting to fit into for years. Perhaps you've always wished for a 24-inch waist, or firmer thighs. It's up to you; set your goal and establish it firmly in your mind. Be sure to set realistic goals.

Second, you should set a target date to reach that goal. If you follow the nutrition and weight-training programs in this book, it is entirely realistic for you to plan to lose one dress size per month. If your dream is to be three sizes smaller, you can set a goal of three months from today. Concentrate on meeting that specific goal.

Third, write a list of changes you are willing to make in your life to reach that goal. Are you willing to commit yourself to weight training six days a week and an alternative form of exercise on the seventh day? Are you going to work on your posture to make yourself look and feel better? Are you prepared to eliminate sugar, fats, and other poisons from your body? And are you determined to spend time each day visualizing your body as you would like it to be?

Fourth, work on your mental attitude to allow yourself to be successful. Start living as though you've already achieved your objective. Begin to see yourself as a successful, competent, and self-confident woman—a woman who can take charge of her health and her body. Be proud of yourself for choosing an exercise program and then sticking to it.

As you follow these steps, you'll notice that you will not only achieve the goals you have set for yourself, but you will then set new goals, and reach those, too.

CHANGE YOUR BODY/CHANGE YOUR LIFE

By conscientiously following the exercise and nutrition programs in this book, we can guarantee that you'll redesign not only your body, but your life as well. You'll have more energy, more stamina, and more strength. You'll sleep better and wake up more refreshed, with greater enthusiasm for the day ahead. We've already explained how your health will improve dramatically.

Your posture will make you *look* more self-confident; don't be surprised if that self-confident look starts to make you *feel* self-confident. Many women who have gone through our program tell us their self-image has improved 100 percent. They're self-assured. They handle problems better (yes, they even become better organized and have less trouble balancing their many roles). That's because, once you begin to take charge of one area of your life, you find it easier to handle the other areas as well. Exchanging your sedentary routine for a healthy, active lifestyle will make you a more enthusiastic, vital person that others enjoy being around.

Remember—YOU ARE IN CONTROL OF YOUR BODY AND YOUR LIFE. But remember too that changes won't happen unless you think about them, really *concentrate* on them, *every day*—and take steps to make them happen. You can change your body! You can change your life!

One of the most effective ways to think your way to a new body is through affirmations. Affirmations are positive statements about yourself and your life. Imagine yourself as you would like to be and then describe yourself in the present tense, with all those attributes achieved.

Close your eyes and describe what you see as you visualize the new you. Don't be shy. Say your affirmations out loud:

"I love to exercise. It keeps me slim and healthy."
"I am slim, strong, and energetic."
"I am feeling light, energized, and fully alive."
"I can accomplish anything I truly want to."
"I see form and beauty in my body."
"I am happy with myself and the world I live in."
"I am exactly what I want to be."
"I am ready to be slim; the fat is melting away."
"Doubt and uncertainty have no power over me."
"I am assured of success."

Write out your own affirmations. They should be strongly positive statements that you repeat whenever a negative thought crosses your mind. Soon the positive attitude will be ingrained in you. Your mental attitude will make the difference in what you accomplish, believe us!

THE SUCCESS JOURNEY

It is natural to find your goals and your own personal definition of success changing as you become more self-confident, more in control of your life. Remember: Success is a journey, not a destination. Those who fail to realize this simple fact are usually terribly disappointed when they reach a goal. Each goal on our journey leads to more exciting goals— goals we can keep achieving. As we journey we realize that each new goal and each new achievement instills a feeling of constant success. And isn't *that* our greatest goal?

HOW TO ANALYZE YOUR BODY

You may be large-boned and voluptuous, lean and muscular, or petite and delicate. Whatever your genetic inheritance, you will look healthier, as well as more attractive and more feminine, if your body is in shape.

Perhaps the most important message in this book is that you can have greater control over your body's shape and fitness than you ever thought possible. You can learn how to alter your proportions, banish dimpled flesh, add curves, and reduce overall dimensions.

In order to design weight-training programs to solve the specific figure problems of the women whose stories you read in Chapter 2, we first analyzed their bodies in terms of body type, height and weight, percentage of body fat, and areas in need of spot reducing. Using these criteria, we were able to plan a program designed to provide maximum benefits in the amount of time each woman could devote to weight training.

In the next chapter, we will present a variety of weight-training programs designed to solve various figure problems. In order to choose the one that's best for you, you will first need to analyze your own body, critically and objectively, keeping those same four criteria in mind.

THE THREE BASIC BODY TYPES

The three basic body types are the ectomorph, endomorph, and mesomorph. Every woman has at least a few traits of all three, but if you read the following descriptions, you'll soon see which basic type you are, and what that means in terms of getting the most out of your weight training and nutrition program.

ECTOMORPHS are usually long, lean, and the least likely to have a problem with overweight. In fact, their complaint is often that they can't maintain their weight. If you're an ectomorph, you should add extra protein to your diet and eat plenty of natural complex carbohydrates. Your training program should involve heavier weights and more sets, but with generally fewer repetitions. You should spend a few extra minutes warming up, because your longer muscles require a little more time to ease into exercise. Greater emphasis should also be placed on exercises for the arms and legs, which usually need to be developed to a greater degree in order to achieve the proper body proportions.

Although ectomorphs are born to be thin, they may have pockets of fat. Remember Eleanor's thighs in her "before" pictures? She was a perfect example of a skinny person with excess fat deposits.

ENDOMORPHS are generally built shorter and thicker, with a fairly long trunk but shorter arms and legs. Their slower metabolism makes it easy to gain weight, so they're often heavier than they'd like to be. If this description fits you, your nutrition program should be light on fats, and your weight training should emphasize fewer sets with more repetitions of lighter weights. You should try to do more exercises for each body part than your ectomorphic or mesomorphic friends, taking care to keep the momentum going throughout the workout, by resting no more than 30 seconds between sets.

MESOMORPHS are the most balanced body type, with good proportions and a tendency toward more curves than ectomorphs and more lean muscle than endomorphs. They are usually well coordinated and fairly athletic in appearance. A well-rounded nutritional program will keep this body type firm and healthy, along with a training program of medium repetitions of fairly heavy weights.

YOUR BEST WEIGHT?

We believe that the bathroom scale should be outlawed. It has created havoc for the American woman, who is enslaved by the tyranny of the scale in evaluating her body. By following our program, the women you met in this book learned that the numbers on the scale don't matter nearly as much as how they look and feel; that the amount of weight they've lost is less important than how their clothes fit and how much energy they have.

Lean body mass weighs more than fat. Two women, both weighing 130 pounds, will look quite different if one has a high percentage of body fat and the other has more lean muscle. The one with the lean body mass will look far thinner than her companion, even if their height and body frame are the same.

SMALL, MEDIUM, OR LARGE FRAME?

To analyze your height and weight, you need first to determine the size of your body frame. Using a tape measure, measure your wrist just behind the wrist bone. If your wrist is 5–5½ inches around, you have a small frame, no matter how much you weigh. Medium frames are those with wrist measurements from 5½ to 6 inches, while large frames are generally those with wrists greater than 6 inches.

PERCENTAGE OF BODY FAT

An increasing number of "experts" are now admitting what weight trainers have known for years—the ratio of body fat to lean muscle is one of the most effective ways to gauge the fitness of your body, telling a far more accurate story than the number of pounds you read on your bathroom scale.

Intrigued by newspaper accounts of various athletes with low percentages of body fat, more and more body-conscious men and women are trying to determine their own ratio of fat to lean muscle. There are a number of methods to determine this relationship. The most exacting is the underwater weighing test, in which you are totally immersed in a tank of water. Since water is denser than fat, a person with a large percentage of body fat will displace more water than a lean person of the same weight. And a fat person will weigh *less* than a muscular person in this test—because this test actually weighs only the muscle in your body. These tests are becoming so popular that many health clubs and spas now have the necessary equipment available for underwater weighing.

Another method uses skinfold calipers, a simple, fairly accurate device to measure your percentage of body fat. They're available at sports and fitness stores, where prices vary widely, anywhere from $10 to $150. Using the calipers, you measure the thickness of folds of skin at specific points on your body. Then, by a mathematical formula provided with the calipers, you calculate your ratio of body fat to muscle. Since at least half of the fat in our bodies is right there under the skin, the caliper findings are usually quite accurate, providing you carefully locate and measure at the correct places. The caliper test, however, is not as accurate as underwater weighing. Consider that on the same day, Anita had a skinfold caliper test, which indicated her body fat at 22 percent, and the highly accurate underwater test, which registered 16 percent fat. But calipers do give you an idea of approximately how much fat you're carrying around, and they are often more accessible than the underwater equipment.

Even without calipers, however, you can get a rough estimate of your body fat with the old-fashioned pinch test. Grab a pinch of skin, just above the side of the waist, between your thumb and forefinger. If the fold of skin is more than an inch thick, you're carrying around too much body fat.

You will find it beneficial to measure your body fat periodically as you exercise and lose weight. Since muscle weighs two-thirds more than fat, significant changes in your body don't always show up on the scale. But calipers or pinch tests will provide dramatic proof of the changes as you redesign your body.

Many women make the mistake of concentrating on losing pounds rather than reducing their percentage of body fat. If you lose 10 pounds without exercising, you are likely to lose 10 pounds of both fat and muscle. But with weight-training programs designed to reduce body fat, you are actually losing the fat and increasing the muscle for a more attractive transformation. Suzette had her body fat tested at various times during the last year. She reduced her body fat percentage from 36 percent to 24 percent, and is shooting for an ideal of 20 percent or less.

Lean body mass not only looks thinner, it is healthier, because when your body has a high percentage of fat, it isn't deposited only on your thighs, hips, upper arms, and all the other places you can see; it also settles around your vital organs, such as the heart, liver, lungs, and kidneys, where it actually impairs proper functioning. A higher proportion of lean muscle to fat also makes sense metabolically, since muscle burns more calories then fat, even in a resting state.

The average American woman has from 30 to 40 percent body fat, which is why many women have bulges—particularly in the stomach, hips, and thighs—even at their ideal weight. To look thinner, you must transform a sizable portion of that fat into lean muscle, which pound for pound has one-fifth the volume of fat. The models in this book all increased their percentage of muscle and decreased their fat, producing the dramatic improvements you saw in Chapter 2.

Women over 50 should aim for an underwater weight of no greater than 27 percent body fat. The ideal body fat percentage for women aged 18 to 30 is 18 to 22 percent; for ages 30 to 50, 20 to 24 percent fat is optimum; 14 to 18 percent fat levels are found in endurance athletes, such as long-distance runners or avid weight trainers.

Some marathon runners, however, have as little as 5 or 10 percent body fat, which can have detrimental effects on hormone production. For women, dropping below 8 to 12 percent body fat is especially unhealthy, because hormones stop functioning properly and menstruation ceases. The production of estrogen and progesterone is greatly decreased, and the body's critical hormone balance is disturbed. A certain amount of body fat is needed for a healthy, feminine appearance. Too little body fat will only make you look haggard and older than your years.

RECOMMENDED BODY FAT PERCENTAGE

Under 30	18–22%
Age 30–37	20–24%
Age 38–45	22–24%
Over 45	27%

TWO KINDS OF FAT

When you're trying to lose weight and trim your body, you just want to lose fat, right? Wrong. Your body has two kinds of fat, and they come in two different colors—brown and yellow. You want to get rid only of the yellow stuff, which is the kind of fat that causes bulges. Brown fat, on the other hand, achieves its color from its rich supply of blood vessels. It accounts for only about 1 percent of your body weight, and is located near your vital organs, where its purpose is to keep those organs (especially your heart) at the proper temperature. How does brown fat keep your body's thermostat regulated? By burning yellow fat, which is actually stored energy waiting to be used. Brown fat knows when to start burning yellow fat by the presence of a hormone in your bloodstream that is produced by your body when you are cold, digesting food, or exercising: You burn up more yellow fat under any of those three conditions.

Cold can increase brown fat activity by as much as 10 percent. Digesting a meal can also turn up the thermostat by another 10 percent, which is why you'd be wise to divide your daily portion of food into four or more smaller meals, keeping the brown fat activity at a constantly higher rate. Exercise is the greatest stimulator of brown fat activity, since it increases the brown fat speed-up from cold and eating. By consciously stimulating this brown fat activity, you will burn unwanted yellow fat faster.

WHAT ABOUT CELLULITE?

Women often ask us about cellulite, those lumpy bulges of fat on the stomach, thighs, and derrière. Cellulite, a term coined years ago by the French, is simply yellow fat, but the tendency for fat to clump in those ugly, dimply pockets is hereditary. Like all fat, those cellulite bulges can be eliminated through proper exercise and nutrition.

Many common foods, such as animal fats and oils, processed sugar, honey, chocolate, dairy products, alcohol, coffee, tea, and hot spices, are "toxic" to slimness, and result in cellulite. In addition, when the diet is heavy in processed foods, the body doesn't properly eliminate the foreign chemicals. Toxic waste is stored as fat, and must be flushed out of the body.

Drinking 6 to 8 glasses of water a day is crucial in eliminating cellulite; it helps cleanse the system. But you'll never rid your body of this fat without exercise. Program I and the stomach, hips, and thigh exercises in Chapter 6 will work to defeat cellulite. In addition, try jumping on a mini-trampoline for at least 12 minutes a day. This stimulates the body's lymph system, which acts like a biological vacuum cleaner, clearing out waste matter in the system. Drinking water helps to flush it away.

Deep massage will also help rid the body of cellulite. Constant, firm pressure for about 15 minutes at the end of your weight-lifting program will continue stimulating the circulation and help loosen and break down the pockets of fat cells. First massage with long, firm strokes over the bulging areas. Then squeeze the lumps gently but firmly with both hands, as if you were squeezing the liquid from a sponge. Next, this time with your knuckles, do more long, firm strokes. Follow your deep massage with a hot shower. If your shower is equipped with a massage head, apply strong pulses of water to the areas you've massaged.

HOW TO CHOOSE A PROGRAM

There are two factors to consider when choosing a weight-training program: the level of training and the specific exercises.

If you're overweight or are not used to exercising regularly, ease your body into weight training with the Beginner's Program appropriate to your schedule and figure goals. After approximately 4 weeks of training, you should be ready to proceed to the Intermediate Program. If you exercise regularly in a gym or aerobics class, spend a week or two on the Beginner's Program, and then proceed to the Intermediate training plan. After approximately 3 months of training, most women can move up to the Advanced Program.

As a basic rule of thumb, when your body is no longer improving in terms of firmness and strength, it's time to proceed to a more advanced program. By the same token, if after you advance you find yourself constantly sore and fatigued, heed your body's warning and slow down.

To select the best program for you, simply look in the mirror. Are your back and upper arms flabby? Does your waist need to be trimmed and firmed? Do you carry saddlebags of fat around your hips and thighs? And have you forgotten what your calves and ankles look like when they're trim? Select the exercises from each program designed for your specific problem areas. It's your choice.

SPOT REDUCING

We aren't going to promise you a new body overnight. But we do want you to know that you will see a definite improvement in firmness and fitness in as little as 2 weeks. In just 4 weeks, you can be one whole clothing size smaller than you are now.

This book contains 4 programs to firm and trim your entire body, but you can also design your own spot-reducing regime, choosing those exercises specifically designed to re-shape problem areas.

Flabby upper arms can be firm again, bulging waist and midriff can be firmer and slimmer. You can lose more inches from your hips and thighs than you ever thought possible. And even if you've had children, you *can* have a flat stomach again. The Postpregnancy Tummy Flatteners in Chapter 6 will tell you how most women can get their tummies back to prepregnancy proportions.

TO GAIN WEIGHT

If you want to gain weight, exercises can still help you reach your goal. Just use heavy weights—as heavy as you can handle without strain—and do fewer repetitions (about half as many as indicated—8 to 12 at most). You will also need to add more protein to your diet to provide the energy needed for the increased activity you're calling on your body to perform. For every hour of training, increase your normal daily protein intake by 20 grams, which is approximately equivalent to 3 eggs or 3 ounces of tuna fish.

A NOTE ABOUT EXERCISE AND PREGNANCY

Recent research indicates that physically fit women with good muscle tone experience easier pregnancies and childbirths. In fact, many specialists admit that they would rather see an athletic 40-year-old get pregnant than an obese 20-year-old. We urge that all women get into shape before they become pregnant. Biologically speaking, the best time to be pregnant is in the 20s, but an out-of-shape body at any age needs special attention. It needs training to develop the strength and energy necessary for a healthy pregnancy and childbirth. We suggest that a woman train a full 6 months, 6 days a week, before pregnancy, and then continue to maintain her muscle tone by training moderately 3 times a week throughout the pregnancy, or until she feels any unusual signs of fatigue. Check with your obstetrician before embarking on any exercise program.

4

HOW TO EXERCISE CORRECTLY

You won't enjoy the full physical and psychological benefits of a weight-training program unless you do the exercises properly. Just as the fire under a pot of water must be turned up high enough for the water to boil, your muscles must be heated properly if they are to convert fat into energy. The more slowly you train, the less heat is generated by the muscles, and the less fat is burned to produce energy. The most common mistake people make is moving too slowly, no matter what type of exercise program they're following.

To shape, firm, and trim your body effectively and efficiently, weight training must be done with rapid, controlled movements, but not so fast that the momentum of the moving weight does the work. Strike a balance. The movements should be smooth, not bouncy or jerky, or you'll increase the risk of injury. To get the most from the exercise, be sure to go through a full range of motion.

Weight trainers frequently use the terms "flex and lift." This means that before exerting energy in any exercise, you should tense (or "flex") the muscle you are working, and then lift the weight. This forces you to concentrate on the specific muscle or muscles, and gives a controlled, smooth motion. By flexing and then lifting, you will achieve optimum results from your workout.

WHY FREE WEIGHTS?

Most of the programs in this book involve free weights: light dumbbells, barbells, and ankle weights, rather than machines. We believe free weights are more convenient, more economical and more versatile than Nautilus equipment or other machines. And, since free-weight programs can be designed to concentrate on specific muscles or muscle groups, they have also been found to be more effective than machines in spot reducing.

With free weights, it's not necessary to get yourself to a gym, or wait in line to work out on complicated equipment. Free weights can be used in your home or your office, whenever you have time.

Because of more concentrated body involvement, free weights also produce increased flexibility and strength, as well as better all-over fitness. With machines, you move a weight along a fixed path, while with free weights the movement reflects natural body motion. There is more control with free weights, so there's less chance of injury.

DON'T FORGET TO STRETCH

Stretching is a crucial part of your weight-training program. There are two kinds of stretching movements: ballistic and static. Ballistic stretches are fast, bouncy, bobbing movements that can cause soreness and sometimes even injuries. We recommend static, sustained movements in which the muscles are slowly stretched and then held in the stretched position for a period of 60 seconds. It takes at least 30 seconds for a stretch to begin to be effective. Whenever possible, we like to stretch with weights to achieve the maximum stretch.

Stretching, when included as part of your warm-up, starts the blood circulating to the muscles you'll be exercising, as well as preparing the heart, respiratory system, joints, and ligaments for the work to come. Stretching also expands the range of motion you'll be able to achieve during your weight-training program.

Some people waste a great deal of time and energy stretching muscles that don't need to be stretched. They also often injure muscles by overstretching them. The flexor group should always be stretched. These include the posterior calf muscles, the hamstrings (leg biceps at the back of the thigh), the obliques (along the sides of the torso), the deltoid and pectoralis muscles (the shoulder and chest muscles), the biceps (front of the upper arm), upper trapezius (neck muscles), and the inner forearm muscle.

The extensor muscles include the anterior tibialis (front of the calf), the quadriceps (front of the thigh), the triceps (back of the upper arm), the latissimus (mid-back), and the posterior forearm. These extensor muscles should never be stretched because they are usually overstretched already by our everyday movements. The front calf muscles, for example, are stretched simply from walking in high heels. The quadriceps are loosened in the sitting position, and those mid-back muscles are overstretched by poor posture, resulting in round shoulders. Extensors must be developed for strength, and also to create a balance with the stronger flexor muscles.

The same 8 stretching exercises we list here can also be done as a warm-down routine.

1. TRAPEZIUS STRETCH

With arms at your sides, hands holding dumbbells, stretch your neck by trying to touch your left ear to your left shoulder. Hold for 1 minute. Stretch the other side, also holding for 1 minute.

2. DELTOID OR PECTORALIS STRETCH

Lying on your back on a bench and holding a dumbbell in each hand, slowly let your arms drop, and hold the stretch for 1 minute.

3. OBLIQUE STRETCH

Holding dumbbells at your sides, stretch for 1 minute to the left, then 1 minute to the right.

4. BICEPS STRETCH

Holding a dumbbell in each hand, twist your hands in toward your body, so that the back of your hand is facing your hip. Hold for 1 minute.

5. FOREARM STRETCH

Holding the fingers of your left hand with your right hand, bend them back as far as possible. Hold for 1 minute. Reverse hands.

6. CALF STRETCH

Stand with your toes on the edge of a step or block and let your heels hang down, as shown. Stretch for 1 minute.

7. HAMSTRING STRETCH

Stand with feet shoulder-width apart. Elevate your left leg on a chair or ledge about 2 feet high. With the heel of the left hand, press the top of the left thigh and bend the upper body forward as shown. Continue to press for 1

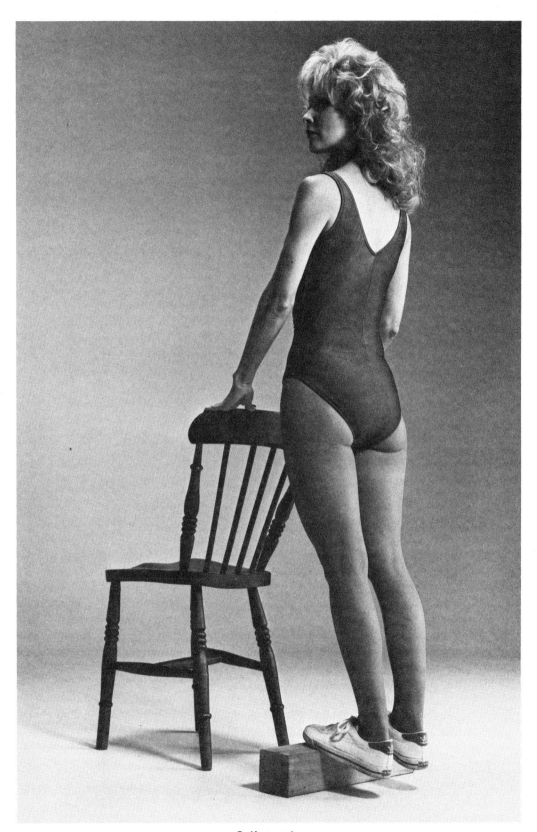

Calf stretch

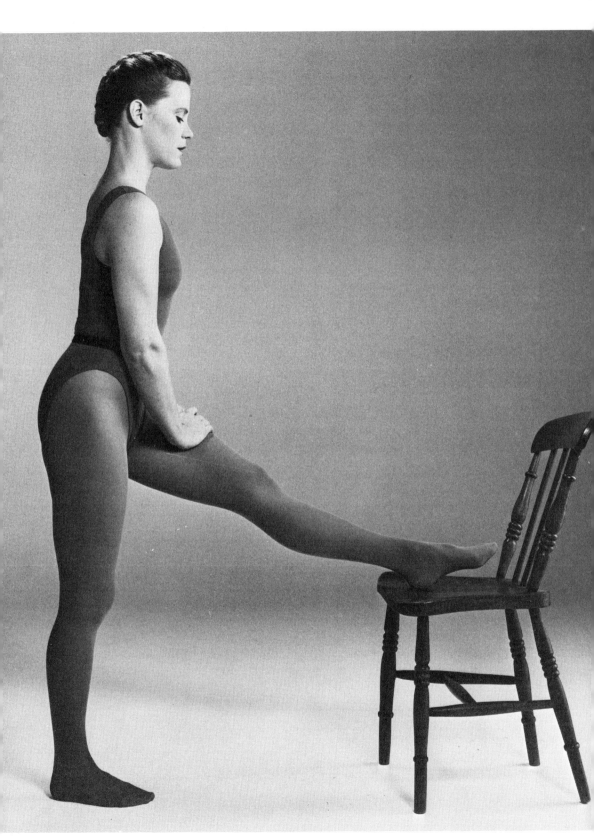

Hamstring stretch

minute, keeping the elbow straight. No extra weights are needed for this stretch, your own body weight provides the resistance.

8. FULL BODY STRETCH

Using a chinning bar, hang from the bar for up to 3 minutes, as shown. Use an overhand grip (see page 47).

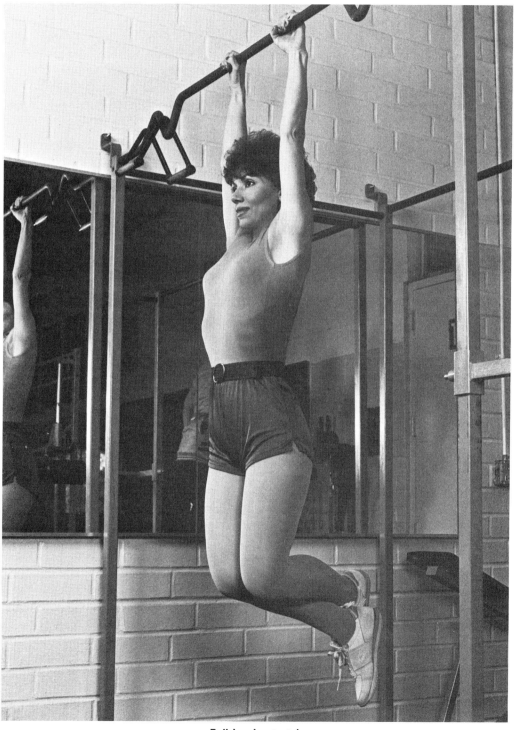

Full body stretch

WARM-UPS ON THE TRAMPOLINE

As you'll discover in many of the following chapters, we are not in favor of any exercise that shocks or jars the body such as jogging or jumping jacks. These movements put unnecessary stress on the spine and joints. Instead we recommend the trampoline or mini-tramp, which cushion the jumps, preventing undue shock to the body.

Combined with stretching, jumping on the tramp is a great way to warm-up and warm-down. Jump continuously for 3 to 5 minutes before and after your training program. Trampoline jumping is an excellent aerobic exercise. We prefer to jump to music, especially some of the livelier songs. Vary your movements as you become proficient on the tramp. You can jump, hop, run in place, practice swimming motions with your arms, or do any other kind of continuous movements that keep your legs moving and your arms and spirits lifted! For a complete aerobic workout, jump continuously for at least 12 minutes.

Another big plus to the trampoline is that vigorous jumping stimulates the circulation and releases glycerol, a natural appetite suppressant, into the system. After about 5 minutes of jumping, hunger pangs vanish. When the munchies hit, head for the tramp instead of the kitchen.

The trampoline is a multi-purpose supplement to any of our weight-training programs. The mini versions are available in fitness stores for under $50. This optional piece of equipment is well worth the investment.

It is important to jump in the center of the trampoline. Jumping near the edge may cause injury since there is not as much spring.

PROPER BREATHING

Proper breathing helps in achieving maximum benefits from your weight-training program. Deep, rhythmic breathing produces more positive results than shallow or spasmodic breaths because it improves circulation, providing working muscles with more oxygen.

Most beginning weight trainers ask when to inhale and when to exhale while doing each new exercise. It's really quite simple:

Inhale as you begin an exercise.

Exhale when you reach the point of greatest exertion.

The outbreath comes when you're asking your body to do the most lifting, pulling, or pushing. Remember to inhale through your nose and exhale through your mouth.

Ideally, you should be breathing fresh, clean air as you exercise. If possible, open a window in your exercise room while you're doing your program. If you work out in a windowless room, stop for a minute several times during your program and go outside for a deep breath of fresh air. Put some bounce in your step, so you don't cool off. You'll feel revitalized and your performance will be better.

NEGATIVE EXERCISES

As in any sport, weight training is always developing new trends. One of them is negative movements. Many trainers teach their students to lift the weight quickly and lower it slowly. We never recommend this kind of movement because it increases the stress on the weakest part of the muscle, its point of insertion. It also forces the muscle to work against gravity and perform an unnatural motion. Muscles are made to lift by contracting, a motion that should be smooth and controlled. The muscle stretches as it lowers the weight. The contraction and stretch should be smooth and evenly paced; with quick contractions and slow stretches, you risk injury to the muscle itself. And in our experience, the results of these negative exercises are inferior to those obtained by traditional movements. Moreover, we find that many of our patients who have tried negative exercises wind up with injuries at the insertion point of their strained muscles. These are difficult to treat, and require a long recuperation period.

PROPER GRIPPING POSITIONS

It is extremely important to use the correct grip for each kind of lift. An improper grip is more than merely uncomfortable, it can result in injuries, dropped weights, muscle strains, and body misalignments. The correct grips are not difficult to learn. Like everything else in weight training, they just take concentration.

UNDERGRIP: Used in exercises for the front upper arm and biceps, in this grip palms are up, with fingers grasping the bar from below. Do not use this grip for overhead lifts.

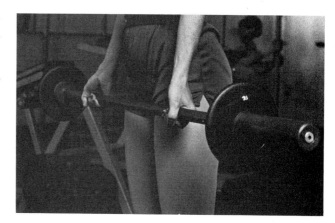

OVERGRIP: Palms face the floor and fingers grasp the bar from above in this grip, which is used for all overhead lifts.

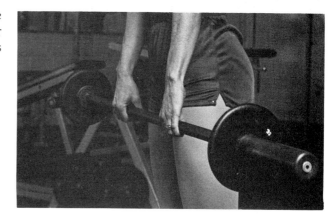

REVERSE GRIP: This grip may be used for heavy lifts and combines the 2 grips described above. With one hand in an undergrip and the other in an overgrip, the weight is usually lifted from the floor to thigh height (as in a dead lift).

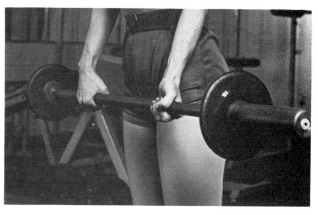

WATCH YOUR FOOT POSITION!

Unless the directions for a particular exercise specifically indicate otherwise, we recommend keeping your feet shoulder-width apart while exercising, with the toes pointing straight ahead. There has been a tendency in recent years to do leg exercises with the toes pointing either in or out, but we have found that by keeping the feet straight you can achieve the same results, while decreasing the chances for injuries. The only exception to this rule is when doing inner and outer thigh back leg raises.

TRAINING PARTNERS

Working out with a training partner can take the drudgery out of your training sessions, increase motivation, and help ensure that you are doing the exercises correctly. As with any partnership, however, it's important to pick your companion carefully.

We recommend that you work out with another woman, because the exercises for men are often quite different from those designed to solve a woman's figure problems, and it's usually easier to train with someone who is doing the same or similar programs.

You should both be at about the same level of competence, with similar commitment and goals. Choose someone reliable, or you'll find your workouts delayed by her tardiness or unavailability. And look for a partner with a similar work and leisure schedule. It's frustrating to have your sweatshirt on, ready for a 7:00 P.M. workout, and find that your partner has to work late at the office again.

Be sure to give each other plenty of encouragement. You may need to coax and push from time to time, but never do so to the point of intimidation. Watch each other's training form carefully, remembering that exercises done incorrectly not only fail to achieve the results you are seeking, but can also cause injuries.

You may also share the expense of training equipment with your partner. In this way, you can either reduce the size of your investment or, by combining resources, you can purchase a more extensive variety of equipment.

Be sensitive to each other's moods, too. There will be times when one of you will be feeling not quite up to par, and you'll appreciate a supportive partner. Give each other understanding and encouragement, and you'll both excel.

On the other hand, you might find that you prefer working out alone. A too-chatty buddy can make it difficult for you to keep your mind on training correctly. And sometimes it's difficult to find someone with a compatible program and schedule. Experiment with partners and working out alone to find which works best for you.

THE DOS AND DON'TS OF WEIGHT TRAINING

The Dos

+ *Do* make your weight training an exercise for your mind as well as your body. Visualize yourself as you would like to be. Concentrate on seeing your arms and legs firmer and stronger, your torso leaner and more supple, your skin smoother and more glowing. Picture yourself healthier, happier, more attractive, and more relaxed.

+ *Do* give yourself positive reinforcement by checking your body each week with a tape measure. You'll see steady progress, and your motivation will soar.

+ *Do* tense your entire body as you exercise, no matter which specific muscles you are working at the time. You'll burn more calories, and every exercise will have a positive effect on your whole body.

+ *Do* experiment with your training schedule to determine when you feel most comfortable exercising. If you decide that the first thing in the morning is best for you, make certain to devote a few extra minutes to warming up your body after its long night's rest.

+ *Do* exercise consistently and try not to miss workouts.

+ *Do* plan to exercise 6 days per week if you want to redesign your body.

+ *Do* set both short- and long-term goals for yourself. Establish new ones as you meet your initial goals.

+ *Do* allow yourself to take pride in each accomplishment.

+ *Do* warm up before every training session.

+ *Do* inhale as you begin each exercise and exhale as you reach the point of greatest exertion.

+ *Do* perform the exercises in the sequence in which they are given. We have planned each program to keep specific body parts moving for the optimum number of sequential exercises. By doing the exercises for the upper body in sequence, for example, you keep the extra blood (and the extra oxygen) in that area, enhancing the effects of all the exercises. Skipping around from exercise to exercise within a program will cause you to lose momentum, and the exercises themselves won't be as effective if they're done randomly.

+ *Do* exercise with a partner, if possible. Watch each other to make certain you're both doing the exercises correctly.

+ *Do* double-check adjustable weights before beginning your workout to make sure that they are secure.

+ *Do* make certain before you begin to exercise that you have all the equipment you need in front of you so that you don't have to interrupt your flow of movement after you have begun your program.

+ *Do* use correct posture when exercising; i.e., for exercises performed in a standing position, keep your spine straight, shoulders level, and weight balanced evenly on both feet—unless the instructions for a particular exercise specify differently.

+ *Do* try to complete your program at least one-half hour before meals, or wait at least an hour after meals before starting.

+ *Do* drink a little water every 10 or 15 minutes while training. Water promotes circulation throughout the tissues of the entire body, making it easier to get rid of all the waste products in the body that cause cellulite.

+ *Do* remember that concentration is crucial in obtaining results with your program. Concentrate on your goals, and have faith in your ability to achieve them.

+ *Do* look at photographs showing the way you'd like to look. They might be photos of yourself when you were thinner, or pictures of someone else. Either way, study them, then visualize yourself looking like that. And then continue your efforts to make it come true, knowing that you *can* succeed.

+ *Do* have a friend take pictures of you as you progress in your weight-training program. Pictures taken at 4-week intervals will show your progress and boost your morale.

+ *Do* keep a careful food diary. (See Chapter 13 on nutrition.)

+ *Do* realize that exercise speeds up your body's metabolism—not only while you're working out, but also for several hours afterward. In other words, your body continues to burn more calories long after you've taken off your sweat suit and put away your weights.

+ *Do* appreciate the value of visualization in reaching your goals. Picturing yourself as you would like to be is vital to making that image a reality. Just as many doctors believe that a patient must have the will to recover in order to do so, you must have the will to be slimmer, firmer, healthier, and more attractive in order to make it happen.

+ *Do* accept the fact that you aren't satisfied with your body as it is. If you were, you probably wouldn't be reading this book. But also accept the fact that you can produce dramatic changes in the way you look and feel, and in less time than you would have thought possible.

The Don'ts

− *Don't* expect diet alone to give you the body you've always dreamed of having. Only a combination of exercise and sound nutrition can produce lasting results.

− *Don't* rest more than a minute between sets, or your body will cool down, the extra blood—and oxygen—will leave the areas being exercised, and you'll lose your momentum.

− *Don't* confuse weight training with the fads and gadgets you've probably already tried in your quest for your ideal body. Weight training is a tested, proven program for all-around health and fitness.

− *Don't* think you have to spend a fortune to get started in weight training. You can get a set of 5-pound dumbbells for $10 or less. A barbell and plates will cost about $35 for a complete set. If you're on a tight budget, check the classified ads for second-hand bargains. Or improvise, using books of various weights, cans, or even your household iron. While a bench with lift and leg curl apparatus generally costs about $60, you can substitute a piano bench or picnic bench from your patio.

− *Don't* think that you must exercise in a gym. In fact, you can probably exercise even more effectively at home, as long as you have a room large enough to allow you to move your arms and legs around freely. At gyms, socializing often interferes with the serious business of improving your body. And it's often necessary to wait to use certain pieces of equipment, especially at peak times, thus interfering with the momentum and aerobic effects of your workout.

− *Don't* exercise to the point of exhaustion. You should feel pleasantly tired after completing your exercises.

− *Don't* exercise if there is any soreness or inflammation around a joint. (If the condition persists, consult a specialist.)

− *Don't* hold your breath when exercising. Breathe correctly, and your exercises will be even more effective.

− *Don't* wear tight or constricting clothing when exercising. A leotard, sweat suit, or shorts and T-shirt are ideal, but on cold days be sure to keep muscles warm and covered.

− *Don't* ask your body to perform movements it wasn't meant to do. The joints, ligaments, tendons, and muscles of the body all have certain limitations, and these must be respected. Listen to your body, and stop as soon as a movement feels uncomfortable.

- *Don't* watch television or talk on the telephone while working out. Concentrate instead on feeling your muscles in motion.

- *Don't* avoid the exercises that are difficult for you. Welcome the challenge, realizing that the difficulty is a clear indication of the improvement you will see very soon.

- *Don't* look at the floor when weight training, or you'll disturb your balance. Look straight ahead, or at your weights.

- *Don't* allow negative thoughts to sabotage your progress. It doesn't matter if you've failed at losing weight before. This time you *will* succeed, because you are actually changing your body's metabolism through exercise.

- *Don't* fool yourself into thinking that you can achieve your ideal body through half-hearted, hit-and-miss efforts. It will take dedication and perseverance to change your body. But you *can* do it.

- *Don't* say that you don't have time to exercise. This book offers effective weight-training and exercise programs you can follow in as little as 10 to 15 minutes a day. Surely you can find that much time when you realize what's at stake: your future.

5

THE PROGRAMS

It's exhilarating to see the pleasure women experience as they watch their bodies change. Most of the women you met in Chapter 2 have gained and lost weight before, as you have probably done. In fact, many have lost weight time and time again, but never saw lasting results. They were on a discouraging seesaw, and got further and further off balance the longer they dieted. They were never able to sustain the weight loss until they began weight training. Now their bodies are not only slimmer, they are better: younger looking, stronger, healthier, and more efficient.

All it takes to bring this kind of pride and excitement into your life is the decision to begin. We admit that this is the most difficult step to take. Your body has fallen into the rut of inaction; it's only natural to resist change. *You* are going to have to make it work.

You have the choice of surrendering to the inertia of the fat cells and doing nothing, or you can take over and change your body. If you don't yet want to take charge of it, read on anyway—you'll be inspired. If you *are* ready to take control, LET'S GET STARTED!

Visualize the way you want to look. If you haven't already done so, take a moment to look through some of your favorite magazines and find the kind of body you want to achieve. Long and lean? Trim but curvaceous? Choose the one that suits your body type. Once you actually start your weight-training program, you will begin to see results so quickly that you'll look forward to each new day's workout. Have a friend take pictures at 4-week intervals and watch how much closer your body gets to the ideal you found in a magazine. You'll know that each movement is making a difference, that each lift is taking you a step closer to your firm, youthful, supple new body.

Remember that weight training is so effective because it's a combination of aerobic and spot-reducing exercise. Aerobic activities are those that get oxygen into your blood stream and into the muscles, especially the most important muscle in the entire body—the heart. Besides burning the fat and producing a firmer, shapelier you, aerobic activities lower your heart rate and blood pressure, while increasing the actual amount of blood pumped through your body. There are many aerobic exercises you can do to supplement your weight training—walking, running, cycling, cross-country skiing, skating, swimming, and dancing—but none of them will provide your body with the slimming, trimming, health-enhancing benefits of aerobic activity plus the specific spot-reduction benefits you get through weight training.

+ *Only weight training helps you burn fat where you have the most to lose.*

+ *Only weight training produces such precise results that you can pinpoint precisely the areas of your body that you want to reduce and the areas you want to build up.*

+ *Only weight training can begin to show results in as little as 10 minutes a day.*

Some cynics say there is no such thing as spot reducing, but the before-and-after pictures in Chapter 2 are proof that they're absolutely wrong. The explanation is simple: The areas of your body that move the most have the least stored fat. Those that move the least have the most fat deposits. For example, because women do a great deal of work with their hands, they often have defined forearms. Their upper arms, which don't get the same workout, become flabby. Likewise, because women traditionally haven't worked their legs as much as men, female hips and thighs are usually layered with fat. By systematically moving specific muscles in a carefully prescribed weight-training program, you will be reducing stored fat, improving muscle strength and efficiency, and actually reshaping, restructuring, and redefining your body.

Whichever programs you choose to follow, it is extremely important to study our instructions carefully and practice the movements in front of a full-length mirror. Exercises that are done incorrectly can cause more harm than good. Get in the habit of using a mirror to check each muscle as it moves. Learn to see and feel the muscles that are being exercised.

Don't try to adapt a man's weight-training program for yourself. The programs in this book have been designed for a woman's body—a body that is very different from a man's. Women store their excess fat in the upper arms, buttocks, and thighs, while men generally carry theirs in their chest or stomach. And with the possible exception of professional weightlifters, women can't—and probably shouldn't—lift the same amount of weight that men can. Many women who train in body-building gyms become too bulky because they use heavy weights, do slow movements, and fewer repetitions (less than 12).

+   *Women achieve the best results (the most firmness and the least bulk) through rapidly lifting lighter weights with more repetitions, more often.*

REPS AND SETS

Before you begin, there are two basic terms that need to be explained: repetitions (reps) and sets. The number of reps prescribed for you is the number of times you actually perform an individual exercise. If you do 10 reps, you lift the weight 10 times in the same manner. A set is a group of reps. If asked to do 3 sets of 10 reps, you repeat the exercise 10 times, rest, do 10 more, rest, and do 10 more.

HOW OFTEN MUST I EXERCISE?

This is one of the questions we are most frequently asked. The answer depends on what you want to accomplish. If you're out to have fun, exercise as often as you want. If you want to maintain your body in its current shape, exercise 3 times a week. But if you're serious about changing the shape of your body, exercise 6 days a week.

We repeat:

Exercise 2 times a week for fun.
Exercise 3 times a week for maintenance.
Exercise 6 times a week for change.

EQUIPMENT

As we've noted, first of all you'll need a full-length mirror. Your beginning program calls for the minimum of equipment: a set of 5-pound dumbbells and a pair of 3-pound ankle weights. That's it. You could achieve your ideal body with this equipment alone and nothing else, simply by doing more and faster repetitions. But by gradually increasing the resistance—working with heavier weights—you will achieve optimum results in the shortest time span. Once you've mastered the beginner's program, you may want to invest in 10-, 15-, and 20-pound dumbbells and a pair of 5-pound ankle weights. Keep all of your weights nearby as you work out, since you'll lose momentum if you have to look for equipment between exercises.

Some of the advanced exercises require an incline bench, which can be purchased at most sporting-goods stores. Look for one with stationary supports to hold weights when they're not being lifted.

REMEMBER—FOR BEST RESULTS:

It is essential that you never rest more than 60 seconds between any exercises. Don't let your body cool down until you've finished your workout.

NOW LET'S GO!

PROGRAM I
(10- to 15-Minute Program)

If you have very limited time but still want to work wonders for your entire body, this program is ideal for you. It provides an upper body workout, while trimming, shaping, and firming the stomach, hips, and thighs. For the first 2 weeks, do not use ankle weights. Then begin using 3-pound weights. Build up until you're doing the complete program 3 times in 15 minutes, and do it 6 days a week. *If it takes you more than 10 or 15 minutes to complete the program, you're moving too slowly to achieve its full aerobic benefits.*

Equipment:
Full-length mirror
3- to 5-pound ankle weights (1 pair)
3- to 5-pound dumbbells (1 pair)

Warm-up:
Stretches on pages 42–45

Exercises:
One-Arm Rowing
Bent-Over Lateral Raises
Lateral Raises
Bent-Over Triceps Extension
Lying Side Leg Raises with Arm Stretched Overhead
Bent-Leg Sit-Ups
Inner Thigh Back Leg Raises
Outer Thigh Back Leg Raises

Warm-down:
Repeat warm-up stretches after completing program.

Exercise 1: One-Arm Rowing

Stand bending forward, with one hand on the chair and a 5-pound dumbbell in the other, feet slightly apart. Pulling your elbow up, raise the dumbbell to chest level, as shown.

Do 2 sets of 20 reps.

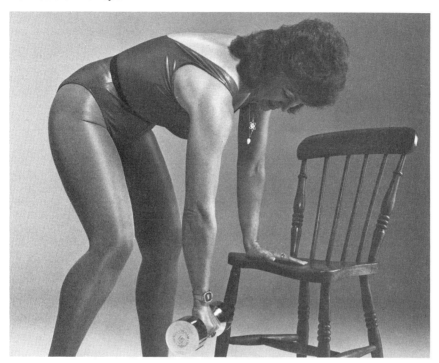

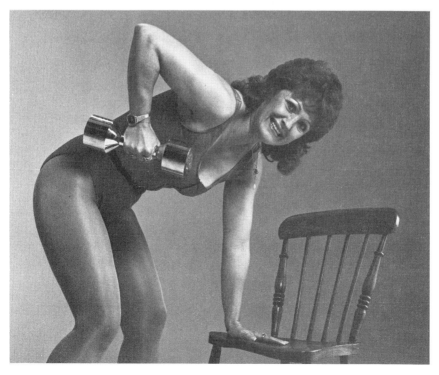

Exercise 2: Bent-Over Lateral Raises

Stand with the feet slightly apart, bending forward as shown, with a dumbbell in each hand. Bending the elbows, raise the dumbbells, then lower them. Repeat.

Do 2 sets of 20 reps.

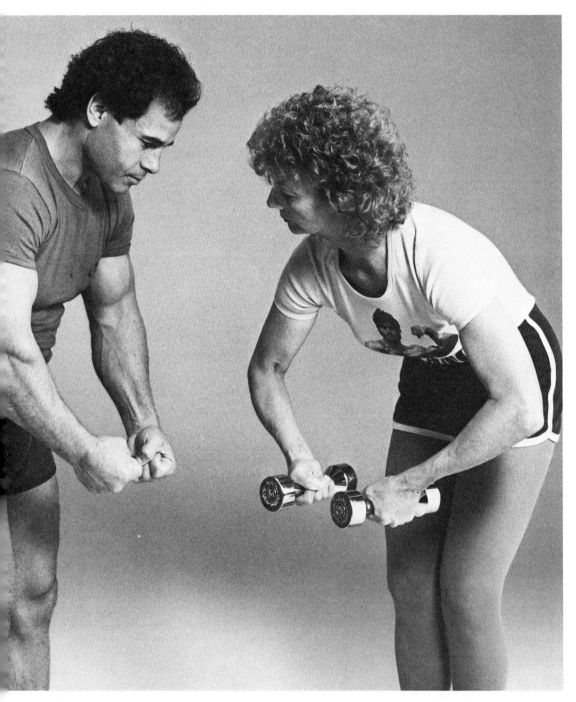

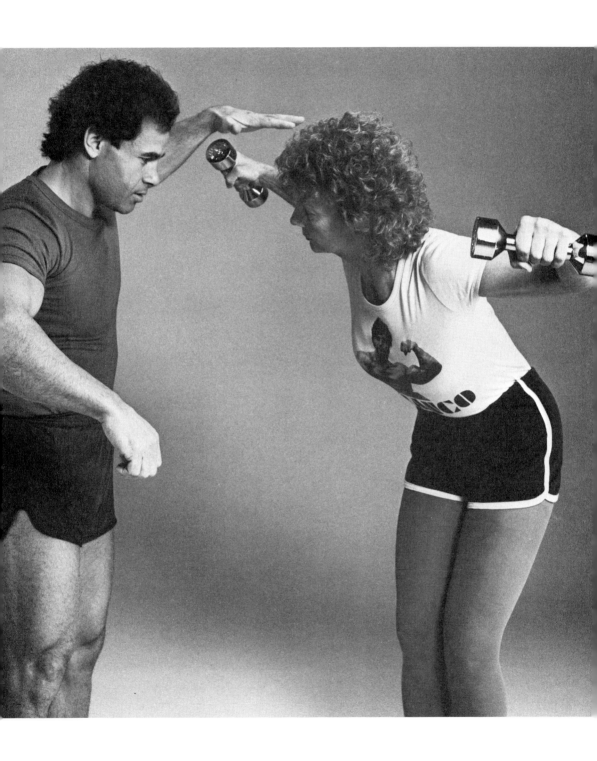

Exercise 3: Lateral Raises

With feet shoulder-width apart and body slightly bent from the waist, hold dumbbells down in front of you. Keeping elbows straight, raise arms to the side until dumbbells are slightly higher than shoulder level. Return to starting position. This can also be done seated, as shown.

Do 2 sets of 10 reps.

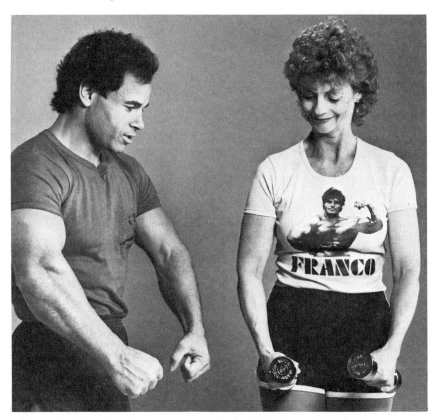

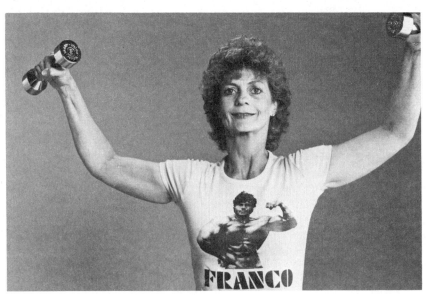

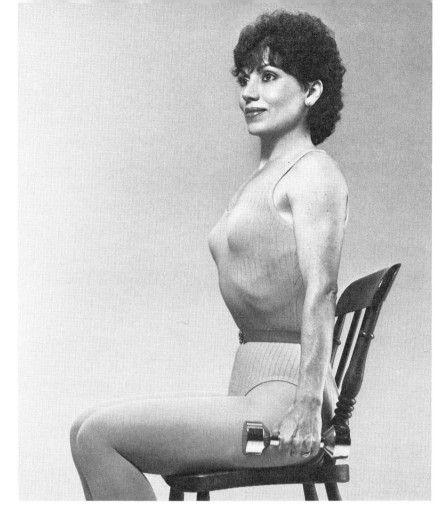

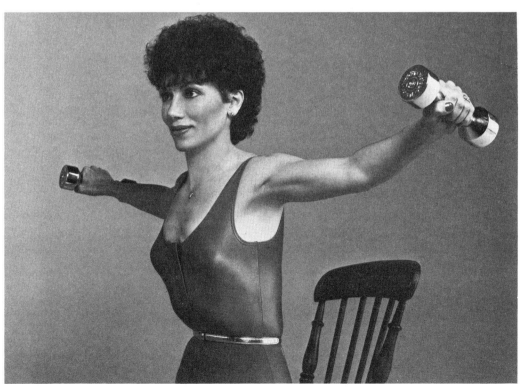

Exercise 4: Bent-Over Triceps Extension

Bending forward from the waist, hold the dumbbells as shown, with arms bent at the elbow. Straighten arms and simultaneously bring them back and up to hip level.

Do 2 sets of 20 reps.

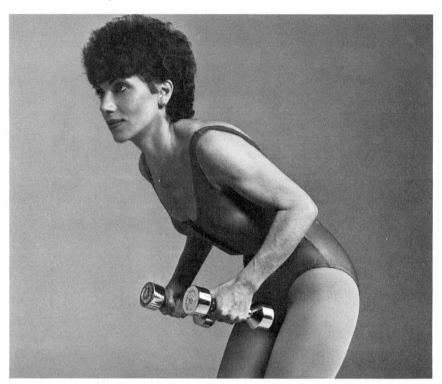

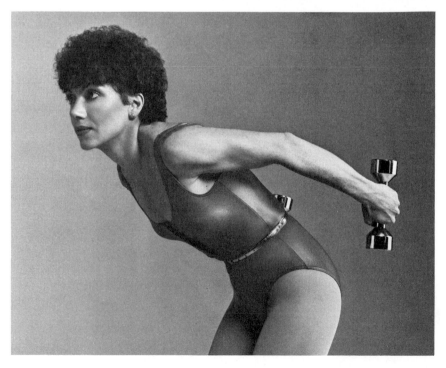

Exercise 5: Lying Side Leg Raises with Arm Stretched Overhead

Lie on your left side, supporting yourself with left arm as shown. Stretch right arm over head. Simultaneously lift right leg and right arm until they meet. Return to outstretched position, making sure to attain a full stretch. When you've completed one set, switch to the right side.

Do 1 set of 30 reps with each leg.

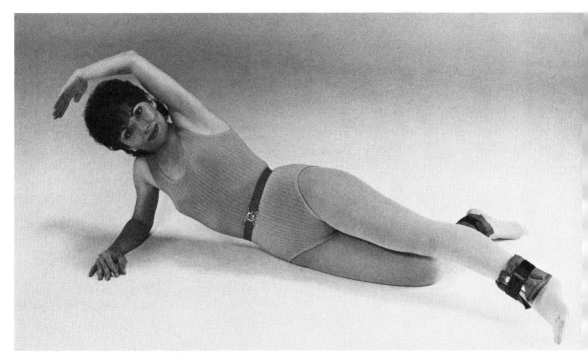

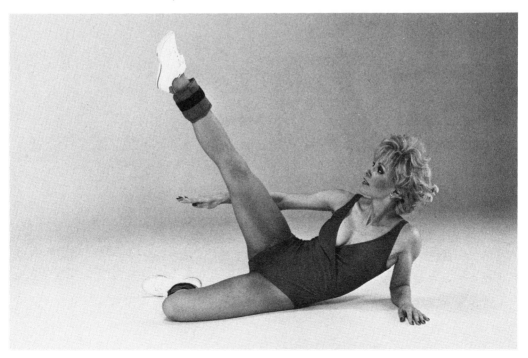

Exercise 6: Bent-Leg Sit-Ups

Lie on your back with your arms overhead and your legs stretched, with feet slightly off the ground. Then bend your knees and bring them to your chest. Simultaneously bring your arms up to meet your knees, lifting your shoulders slightly off the ground but keeping your spine flat on the floor. Then return to starting position and repeat as rapidly as possible. Your abdominal muscles are getting a workout.

Do 1 set of 20 reps.

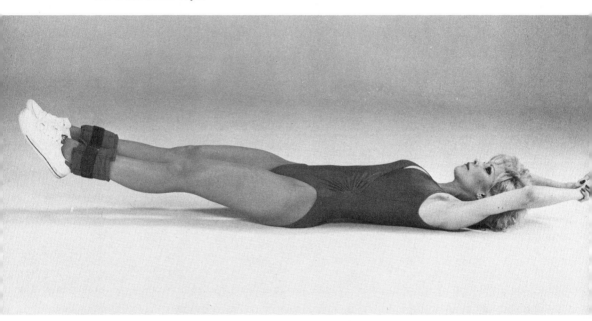

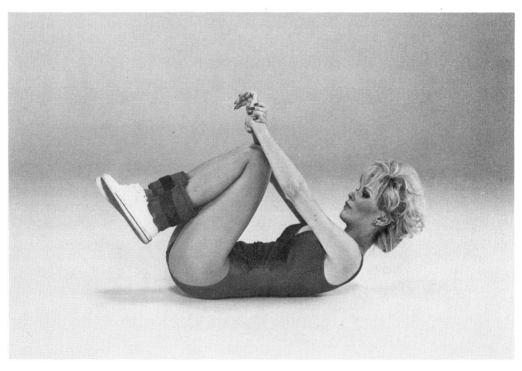

Exercise 7: Inner Thigh Back Leg Raises

On your hands and knees as shown, extend your right leg, flex your right foot, and point your toes in, toward your other leg. Raise your leg as high as possible while keeping your leg tensed. Lower your leg.

Do 1 set of 20 reps.

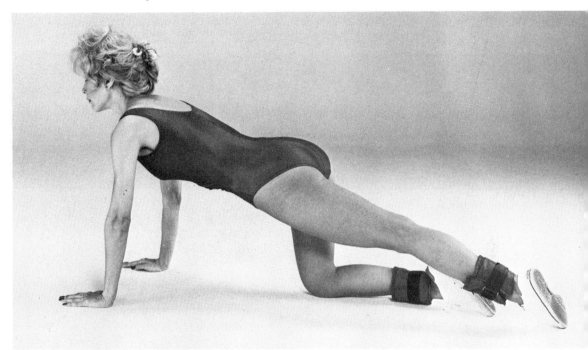

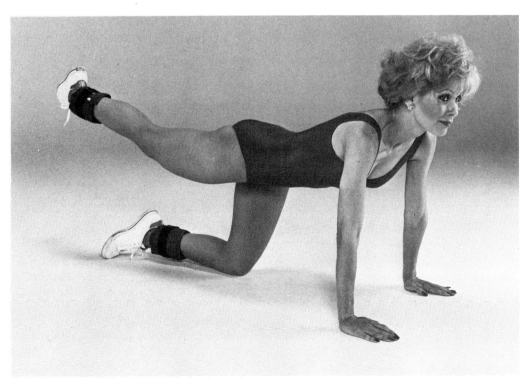

Exercise 8: Outer Thigh Back Leg Raises

Assume the same position as above, but point the toe outward, away from your other leg.

Do 1 set of 20 reps.

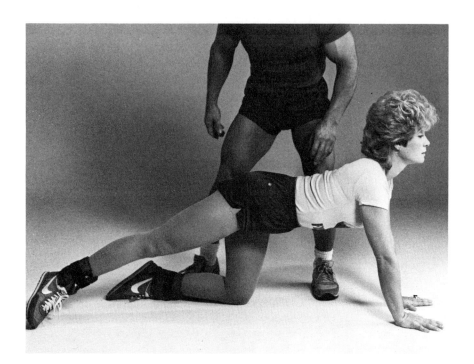

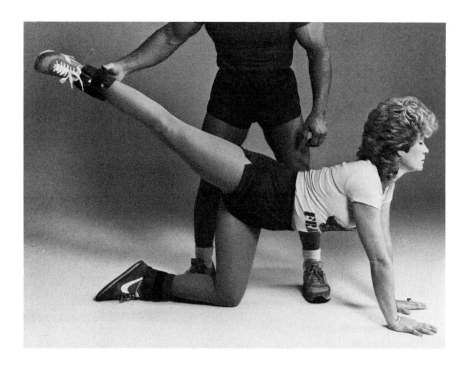

PROGRAM II

(15- to 20-Minute Program)

This program serves as the second stage in all-over conditioning, firming, toning, and trimming. It utilizes the total body workout from Program I, but adds upper and lower body exercises that are slightly more strenuous, making this the next challenge for those ready for further progress. Most women should be ready for this program two weeks after first beginning their weight-training program.

Equipment:
Full-length mirror
Two 3- to 5-pound ankle weights
Two 3- to 5-pound dumbbells

Warm Up:
Stretches on pages 42–45

Exercises:
Standing Overhead Dumbbell Raises
Standing Side Leg Raises

Plus all exercises from Program I, using ankle weights.

Warm-down:
Repeat warm-up stretches after completing program.

Exercise 9: Standing Overhead Dumbbell Raises

Standing and holding a 5-pound dumbbell in each hand at shoulder level, press the weights up over your head.

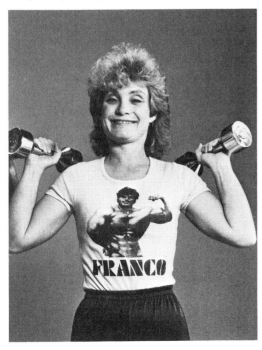
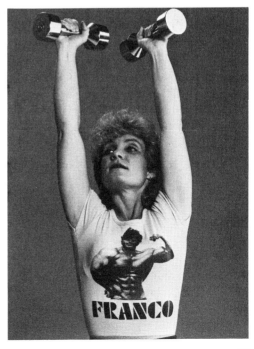

Exercise 10: Standing Side Leg Raises

Stand erect and hold onto the back of a chair. Extend your leg straight out to the side and lift.

Do 1 set of 20 reps.

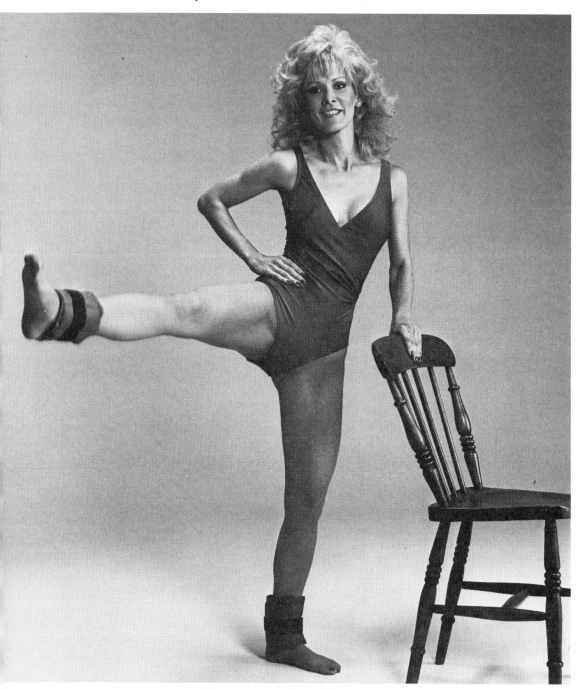

PROGRAM III
(25- to 45-Minute Program)

The incorporation of more advanced exercises plus addition of heavier ankle weights makes this program the third level in weight training, which you should be able to reach after 4 weeks. You'll see steady results with this program, particularly in the hips and thighs, which are effectively whittled by the lunges.

Equipment:
Full-length mirror
Two 5-pound ankle weights
Two 5-pound dumbbells

Warm-Up:
Stretches on pages 42–45

Exercises:
Standing Anterior/Posterior Arm Raises
Dumbbell Curls
Lunges

Plus all of Program I, using five-pound ankle weights.

Warm-down:
Repeat warm-up stretches after completing program.

Exercise 11: Standing Anterior/Posterior Arm Raises

Stand erect with a 5-pound dumbbell in each hand. Swing each hand forward and back as shown in the illustration, for a count of 20 reps with each hand.

Do 3 sets of 20 reps.

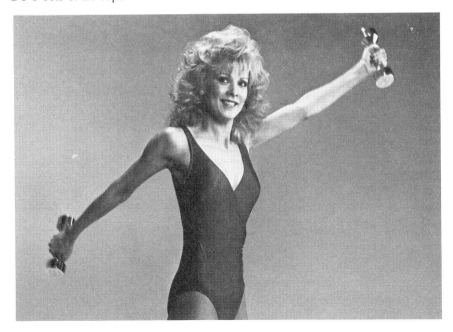

Exercise 12: Dumbbell Curls

Stand with your feet shoulder-width apart and a dumbbell in each hand. Turn your hands so that your palms are facing inward, then, as you bend your arms and bring the weights upward, turn your hands until your palms are facing up. Lower the dumbbells to the original position.

Do 2 sets of 10 reps.

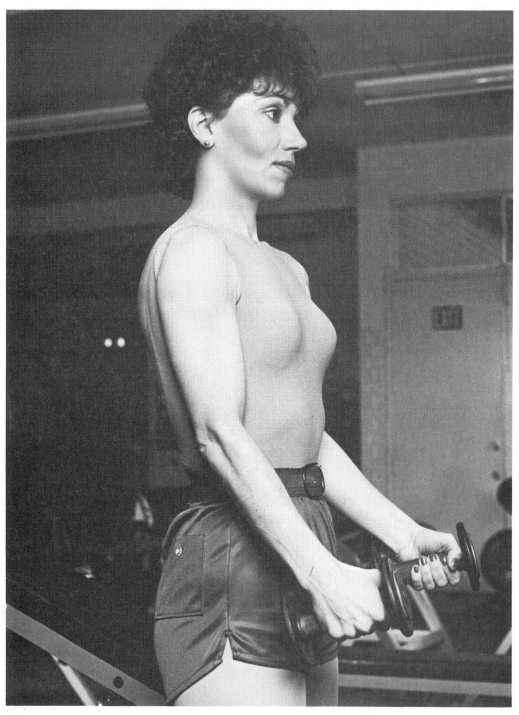

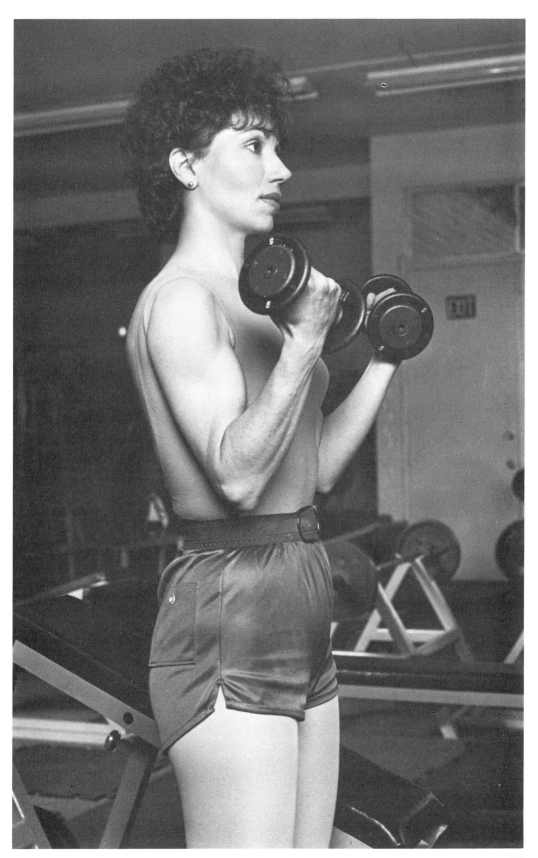

Exercise 13: Lunges

With a 10-pound dumbbell in each hand, stand straight with your feet shoulder-width apart. Keeping your right foot in place, step forward as far as you comfortably can with your left foot, moving your torso down and forward as you do so. Keeping your head and body straight, return to the original position. Repeat with the alternate foot stepping forward. You can also do this exercise with a barbell held behind your neck, as shown.

Do 3 sets of 20 reps

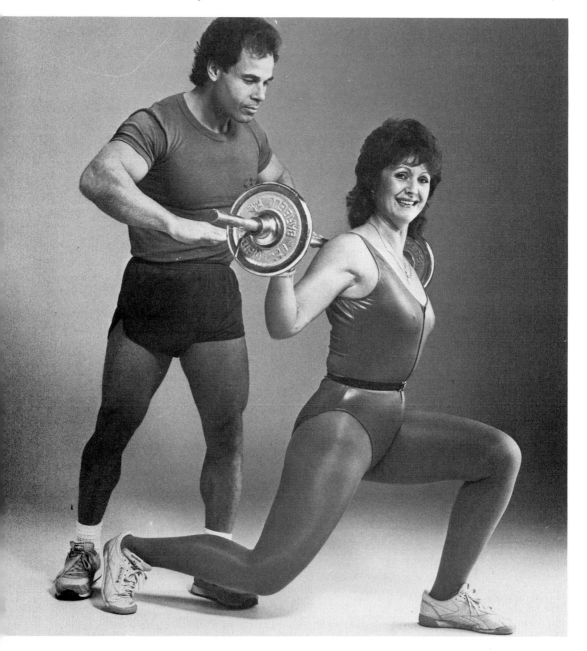

PROGRAM IV
(40- to 60-Minute Program)

This program is for the intermediate weight trainer who has developed strength, flexibility, and endurance. By the time you are ready for this program, which should be within 2 to 2½ months from the day you began training, you will probably have lost at least 2 or 3 dress sizes, and more inches than you had thought possible. In this program, you will be adding upper body exercises to your workout, firming and toning the upper arms, shoulders, and back. When you do the upper body exercises from Program I, use 10-pound dumbbells. The use of 5-pound ankle weights and the addition of barbell squats will enhance the good results you're already seeing in your lower body.

Equipment:
Full-length mirror
Two 5-pound ankle weights
Two 10-pound dumbbells
Bar with 30 to 40 pounds in weights
Bench that inclines

Exercises:
Incline Bench Press
Incline Cross Flies
Barbell Rowing
Lunges
Barbell Squats

Warm-Up:
Stretches on pages 42–45

Plus all of Program I, using 5-pound ankle weights

Warm-down:
Repeat warm-up stretches after completing program.

Exercise 14: Incline Bench Press

Begin by lifting the barbell from the stationary support or from your training partner. If you have neither, hold the barbell across your legs as you sit back against the incline bench. Bring the barbell to chest height, but no higher. Exhale as you push the barbell up until your arms are straight, inhale as you lower it to your chest.

Do 4 sets of 10 reps.

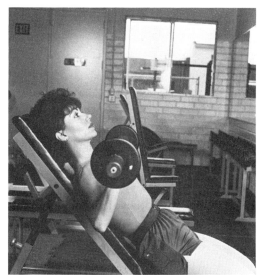
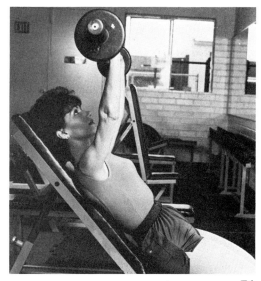

Exercise 15: Incline Cross Flies

With the bench in the incline position and using dumbbells in each hand, begin as shown in the illustration. With elbows bent, inhale and lift dumbbells straight up, crossing your arms after they are fully extended as shown, exhaling as you do so. Uncross and bring your arms back to your side.

Do 3 sets of 10 reps.

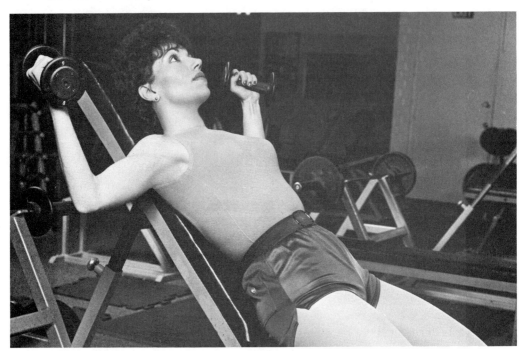

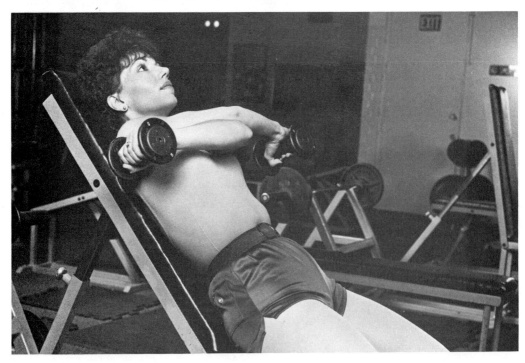

Exercise 16: Barbell Rowing

Bending from the waist, grasp the bar with the palms down, as shown in the illustration, and let the bar hang parallel with your chest and the floor. Bring it up to your chest while you inhale and lower it as you exhale. Repeat.

Do 3 sets of 10 reps.

Lunges

See Exercise 7 on page 63 for description.

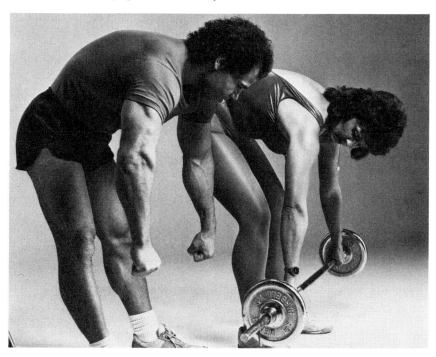

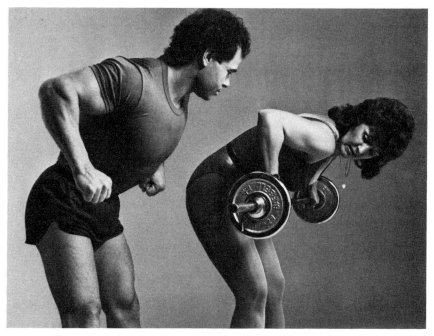

Exercise 17: Barbell Squats

Stand with feet shoulder-width apart, with heels resting on a block or book, about 2 or 3 inches high. With barbell resting on the backs of your shoulders, bend your knees and lower your body as shown. Be sure that the bar is resting on your shoulders, not on the bone at the base of your neck. This is the seventh cervical vertebrae, which is often injured from constant jarring by the bar.

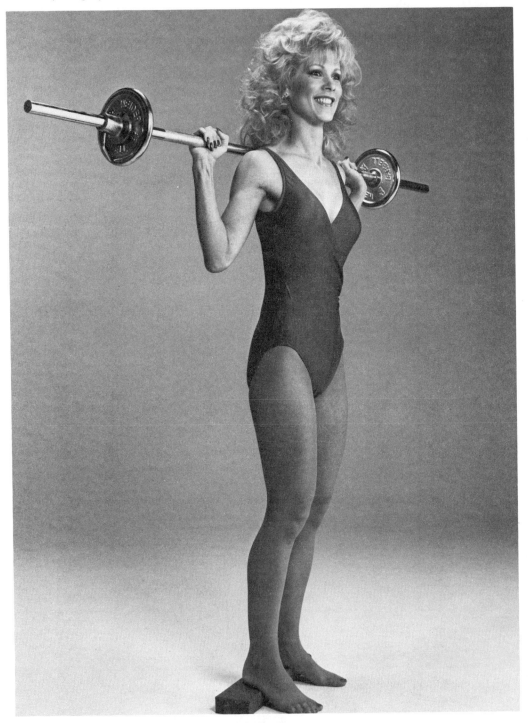

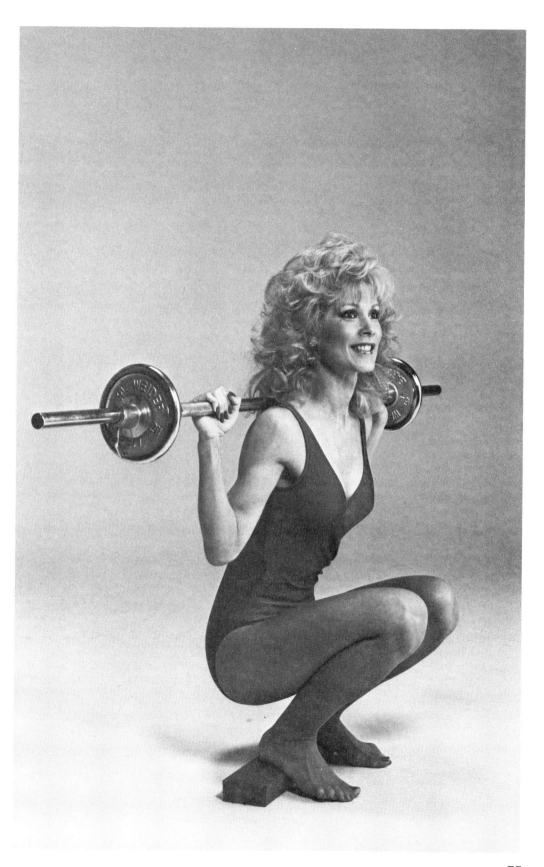

6

SPOT REDUCING

Every body has its trouble spots, those stubborn bulges that women often find more disturbing than their excess weight. In a recent survey, 72 percent of the women responding said they were dissatisfied with their thighs, 64 percent with their stomachs, and 61 percent with their hips.

One of the most exciting aspects of weight training is the freedom it gives you literally to reshape various parts of your body. Chubby thighs, flabby upper arms, and protruding tummies are soon transformed by spot-reducing programs. In fact, training with weights is the only way we know of to reduce, tone, or build up isolated areas of your body.

Following are machine and free-weight exercises for each area of the body. After your basic training program, do at least 3 within each section pertaining to your specific figure problems. With dedicated effort, you should begin to see noticeable improvement in as little as two weeks, and definite changes in your body configuration within a month.

TRICEPS

One of the first signs of aging in women appears in the upper arms, which begin to get flabby and crepey. If you want to look your best in sleeveless blouses and swimwear, pick at least 3 of these exercises to do 5 times a week. For best results, do 3 sets of 20 reps of each.

Exercise 18: Triceps Pushdowns

Stand on the floor in front of the machine. Reach up and grasp the bar with an overhand grip. Keep elbows in tight, touching the sides of the body, and pull the bar down until it is at chest height. Raise, and then pull down.

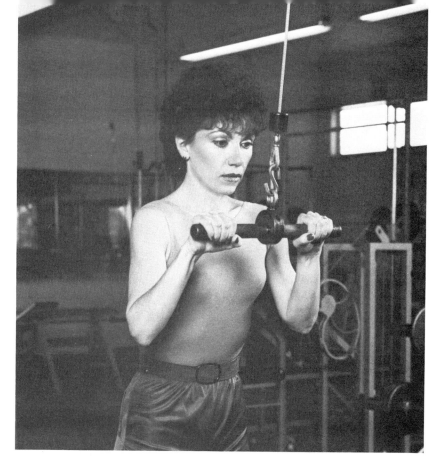

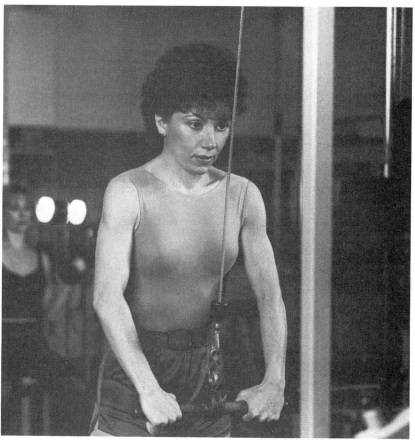

Exercise 19: Lying Triceps Extension

Lying on your back with arms up and elbows bent as shown, lift the barbell up and down toward your forehead. Try not to move your elbows out of position.

Bent-Over Triceps Extension

See Exercise 4 on page 60 for description.

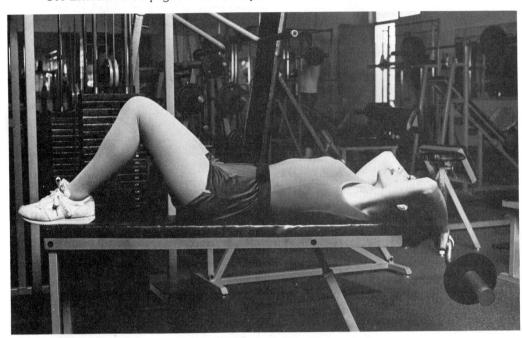

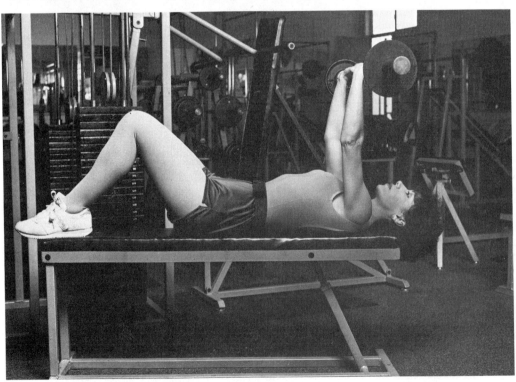

Exercise 20: Seated Triceps Extension

Seated on a bench or chair, hold a dumbbell behind your head at the position shown in the illustration. Straighten the arm over your head and then return it to the starting position.

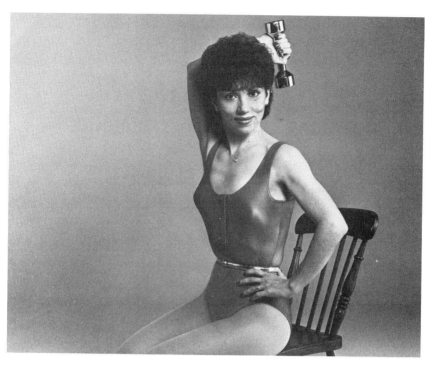

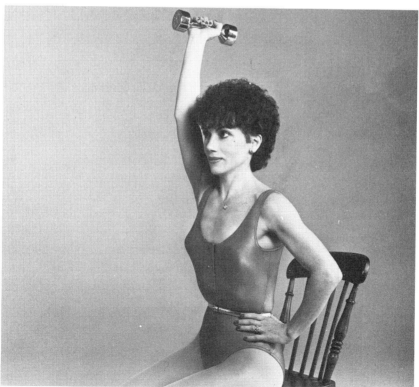

Exercise 21: Triceps Push-Ups

Stand in front of a chair with arms leaning on the seat, shoulder-width apart. Extend legs as shown. Bend elbows and lower body to chair. With a regular push-up motion, lower your body as you bend your arms and push up as you straighten them.

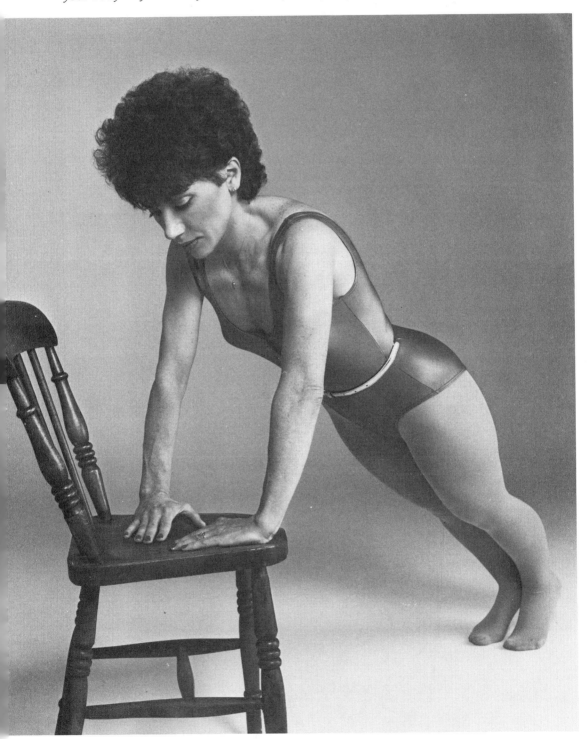

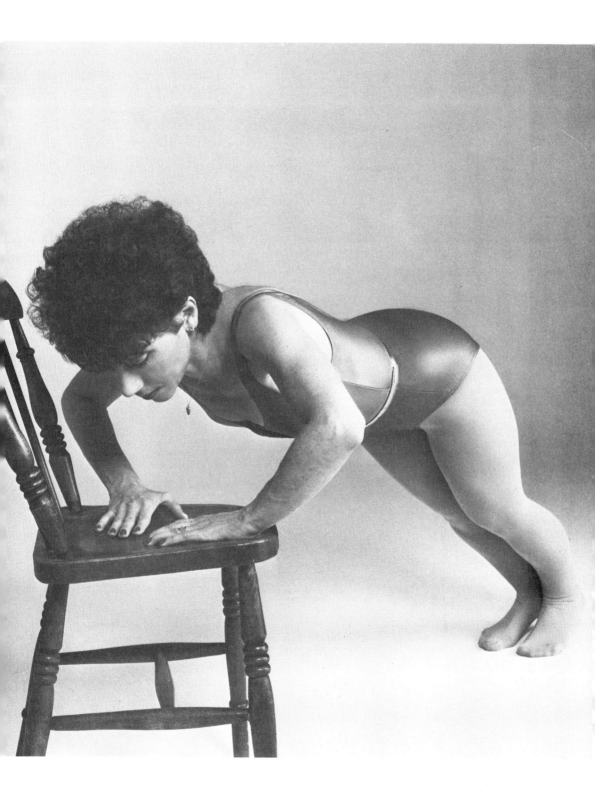

DOWAGER'S HUMP

Many women begin to develop round shoulders even while still quite young, owing to weak shoulder and back muscles. To correct this, you must build up those back muscles, particularly across the shoulders. Pick at least 3 of the following exercises, and do 3 sets of 15 reps, 4 times a week.

Exercise 22: Pulldowns Behind the Neck

In the gym, kneel on the floor facing the pulldown machine and grasp the bar behind your neck with an overhand grip, with your hands about 3 feet apart. Pull the bar down as far as you can, exhaling as you do so. Inhale as you raise, then pull down again.

Exercise 23: Behind the Neck Press

This exercise can be done using the neck press machine, or you may do it with a barbell. Seated on a bench, with barbell resting at shoulder level on the support, lower the bar to your shoulders, then quickly press it up, above your head. Do your reps without stopping between sets. Try to hold your back perfectly straight, and be sure the bar doesn't jar the back of your neck. It should touch your shoulders, not your neck.

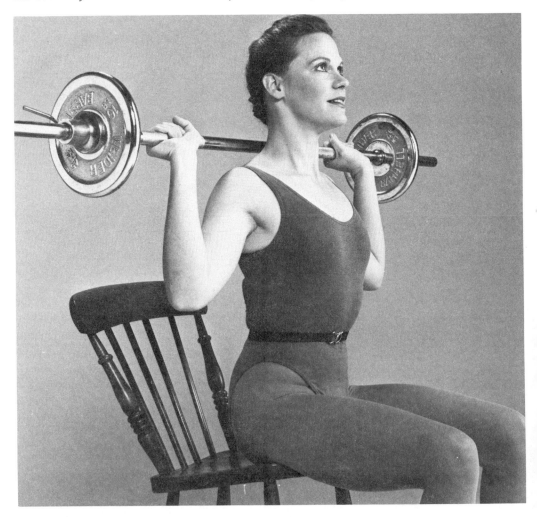

Bent-Over Lateral Raises

See Exercise 2 on page 56 for description.

Exercise 24: Neck Flexion and Extension

Sit or stand straight. Try to touch your chin to your chest. Then pull your head back so you can look at the ceiling.

Do 3 sets of 10 reps.

Exercise 25: Lateral Neck Bends

Stand or sit straight. Try to bring left ear to left shoulder without lifting your shoulder. Return to center. Then try to touch right ear to right shoulder. Return to center. Repeat complete movement.

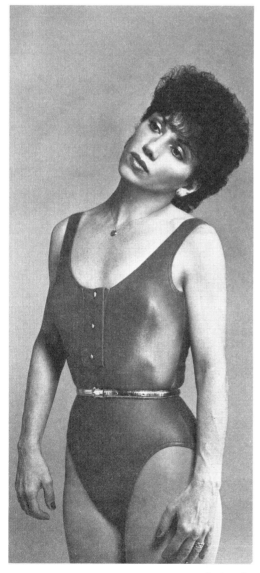 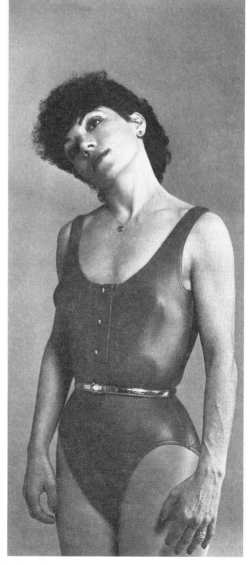

Lateral neck bends

STOMACH, HIPS, THIGHS, KNEES

These spot-reducing exercises are for the stomach, hips, and inner and outer thigh areas. They are most effective when done with 3-pound ankle weights. Begin with no weights, and after about 2 weeks add the 3-pound weights. You will achieve the best results if you do 4 exercises from each group 6 times per week. Begin with 3 sets of 20 reps for each leg exercise and increase to 5 sets of 20 reps.

Stomach

We have divided the exercises for this problem area into two parts: the abdomen and the sides of the waist. Depending upon your particular figure, you may want to use one or both groups. You may be surprised to notice that the traditional sit-up, so often relied upon to firm the abdomen, is not included. We have found that it places too much strain on the lower thoracic and lumbar regions of the spine, so we recommend the bent-leg sit-up instead.

For the Abdominals:
Bent-Leg Sit-Ups
    See Exercise 6 on page 62 for description.

Exercise 26: Bent-Leg Raises

Lie on your back with your arms at your sides, palms down. Begin with your legs straight and your feet slightly off the floor. Bending your knees, bring them to your chest, then straighten your legs, pointing your toes toward the ceiling. Lower the legs to the starting position, and repeat. Do not allow your feet to rest on the floor at any time during the exercise. If your lower back feels strained, place your hands under your hips.

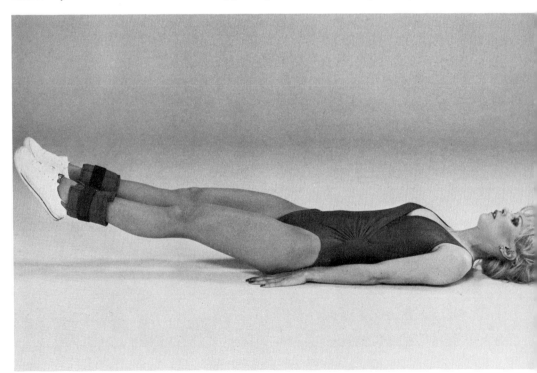

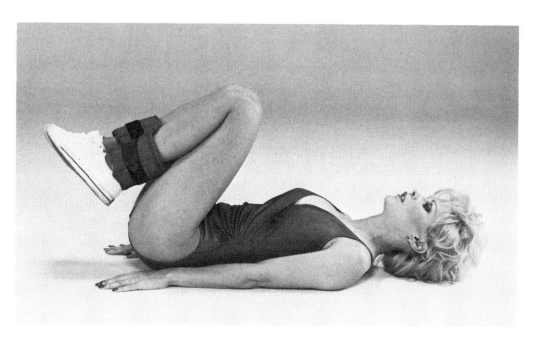

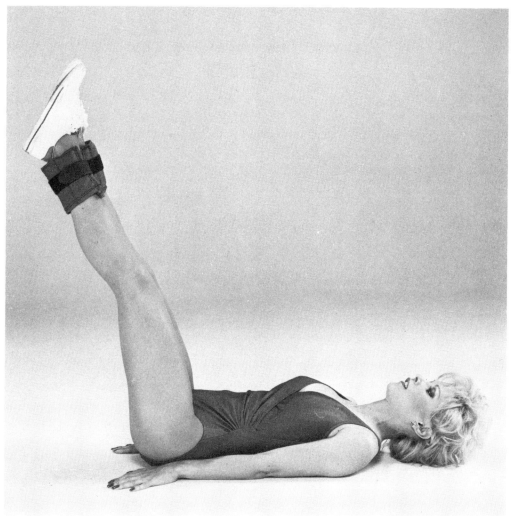

Exercise 27: Straight-Leg Raises

Lie on the floor, with arms at your sides, palms down, feet slightly off the floor. Keeping your knees straight and your legs together, raise them to a vertical position as shown. Lower. If your lower back feels strained, place your hands under your hips.

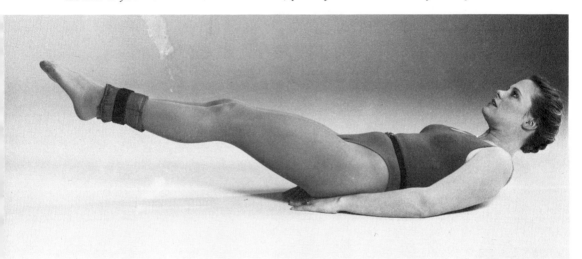

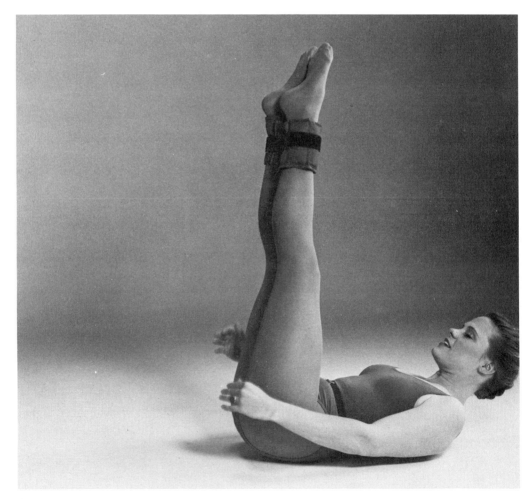

Exercise 28: Alternating Leg Raises

Do this exactly like the preceding exercise, but raise the legs alternately, with carefully controlled movements. Be sure the lowered leg never touches the floor.

Exercise 29: Elbow to Knee

Lie on your back with legs outstretched ready for a bicycling motion. Feet should be slightly off the ground. With shoulders slightly off the ground and hands positioned as shown, touch opposite elbow to opposite knee as you "pedal" at a rapid pace. Be sure to bring knees as close to chest as possible. Important: Do not pull on the head or neck with your hands.

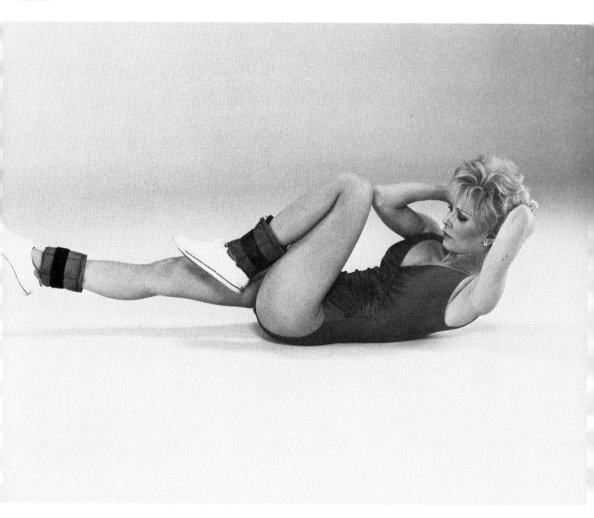

Exercise 30: Crunches

This exercise achieves everything sit-ups should, without strain on your lower back. Lie on your back on the floor, with your legs bent and resting on a chair, as shown. With your arms crossed over your chest, pull your shoulders up toward your knees as far as possible, and then return to starting position.

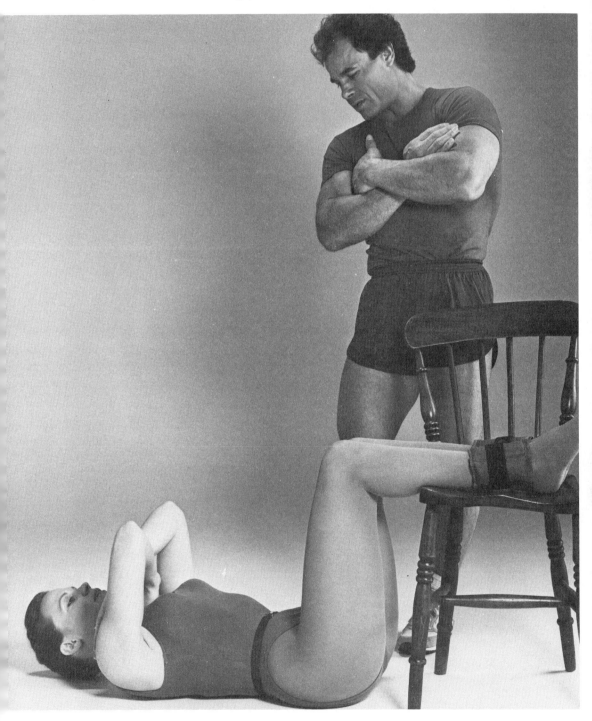

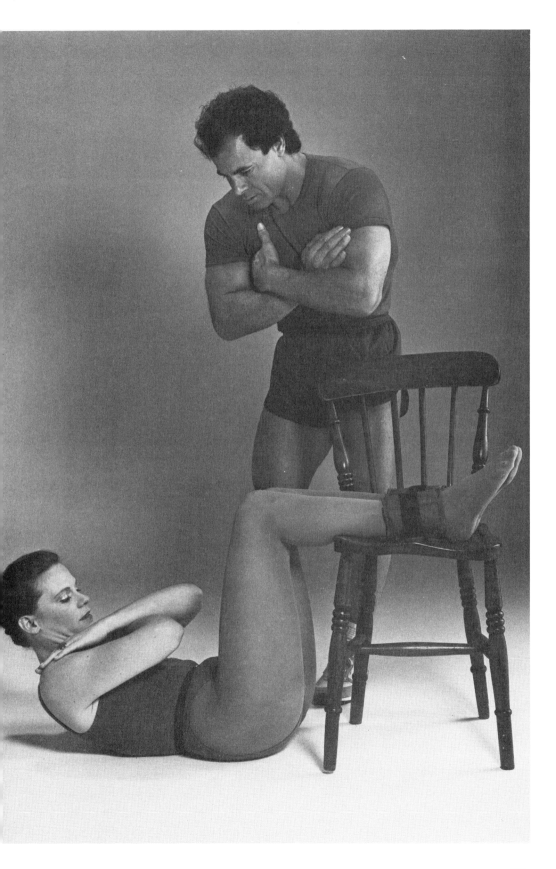

Exercise 31: Straight-Leg Scissors

Lying on your back, with legs in the air and feet together, spread the legs as far apart as possible, then return to starting position. Be sure to keep muscles tensed as you perform this scissors-like motion. If your lower back feels strained, place your hands under your hips.

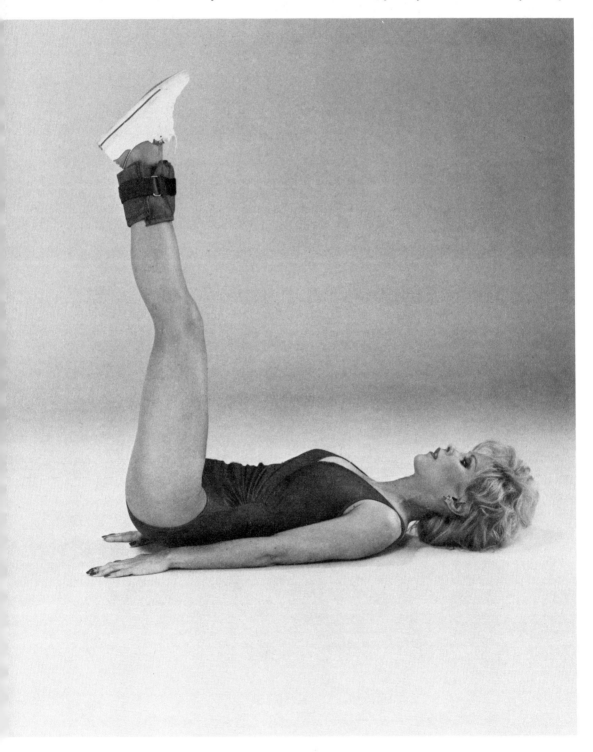

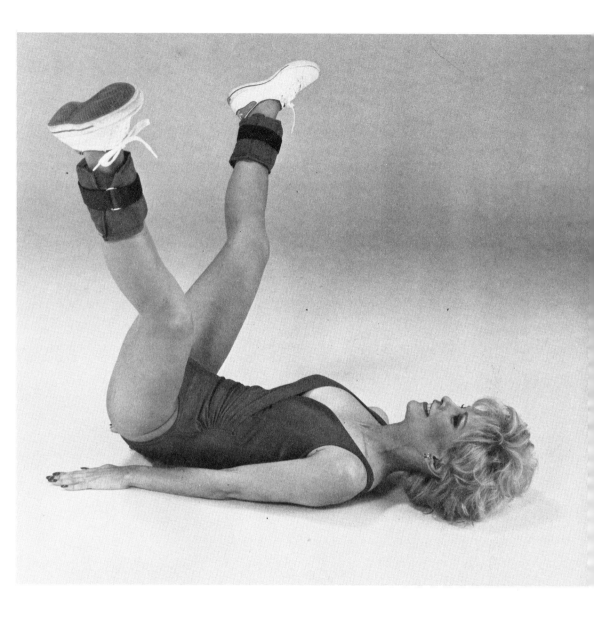

For the Sides of the Waist ("Love Handles"):

Exercise 32: Side Bends

Standing with hands on hips, bend first to the left side, then return to center. Bend to the right and return to center. Count this entire movement as one repetition. *Do not use weights.* It's a common mistake to hold dumbbells during this exercise. Weights will build muscle and width at the waist.

Lying Side Leg Raises with Arm Stretched Overhead
See Exercise 5 on page 61 for description.

Standing Side Leg Raises
See Exercise 10 on page 66 for description.

Thighs (Front and Inner)

Exercise 33: Cable Inner Thigh (Cable Cross)

In the gym, stand with side to the cable machine and attach the cable to the ankle closest to the machine. With a smooth, controlled movement, cross the leg with the cable in front of the other, as shown.

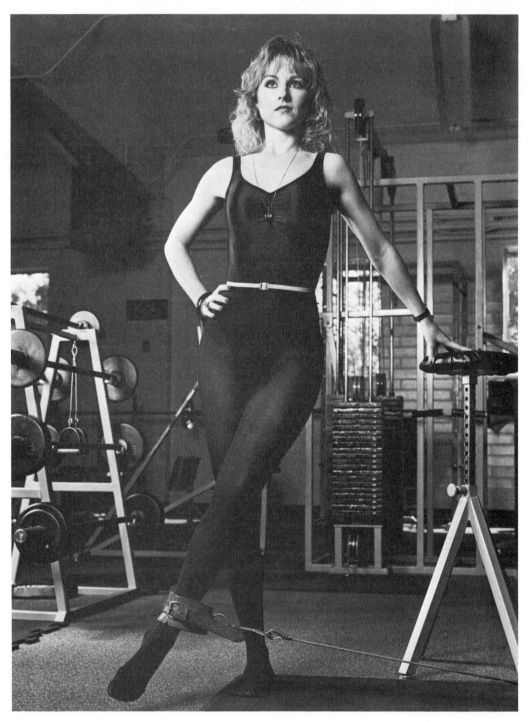

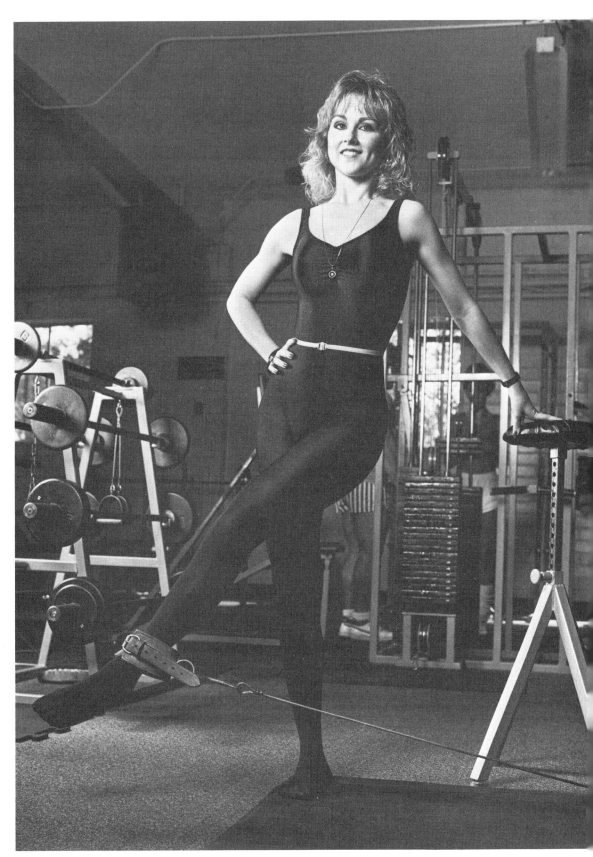

Exercise 34: Lying Inner Thigh Leg Raises

Lying on your right side with left leg bent behind the right leg for support, as shown, support your upper body on your right elbow. With foot flexed, lift the right leg. Lower, and repeat rapidly. Then switch sides.

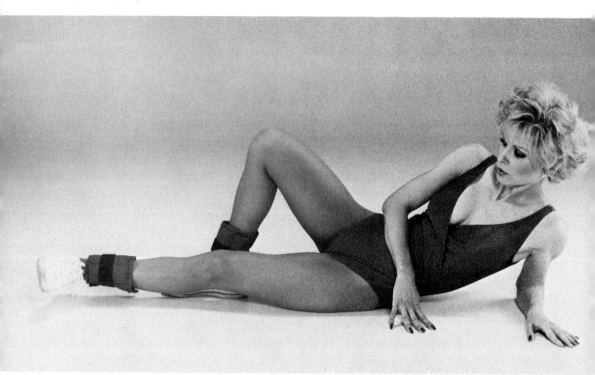

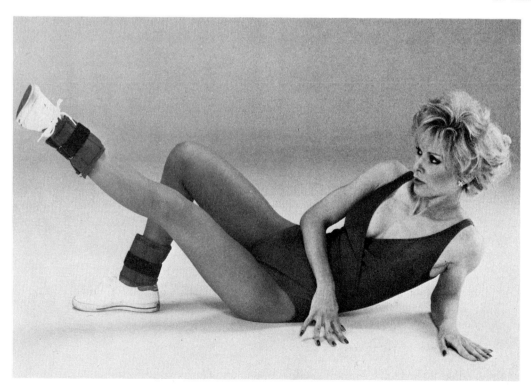

Exercise 35: Standing Inner Thigh Raises

Holding on to the back of a chair for support, as shown, begin with feet slightly apart. Cross the left leg in front of the right, then return to starting position and lift leg out to the side. This should be done in a continuous sweep. Repeat all sets with one leg, then switch to the opposite leg.

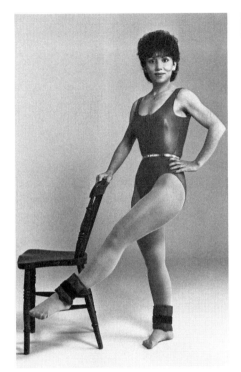 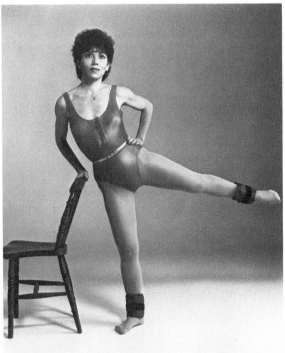

Lunges
See Exercise 13 on page 70 for description.

Exercise 36: Dumbbell Squats

Standing with your feet slightly apart, heels on a 2- or 3-inch block or book, dumbbells held at your side as shown, bend your knees and squat until your thighs are parallel with your knees. Stand up; repeat, using 5- or 10-pound weights.

Barbell Squats
See Exercise 17 on page 74 for description.

Exercise 37: Leg Extensions

This exercise can be done on a machine. See Exercise 70 on page 134 for description. It can also be done at home with dumbbells. To do the exercise with a dumbbell, sit on a bench or chair, with hands as shown. Begin with knees bent and a 5-pound weight held between your feet, which should be resting slightly off the floor. Straighten legs as shown, then return to beginning position. Repeat.

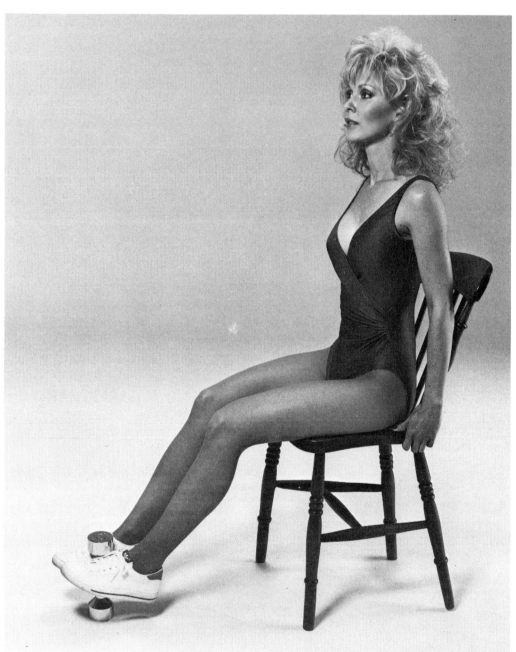

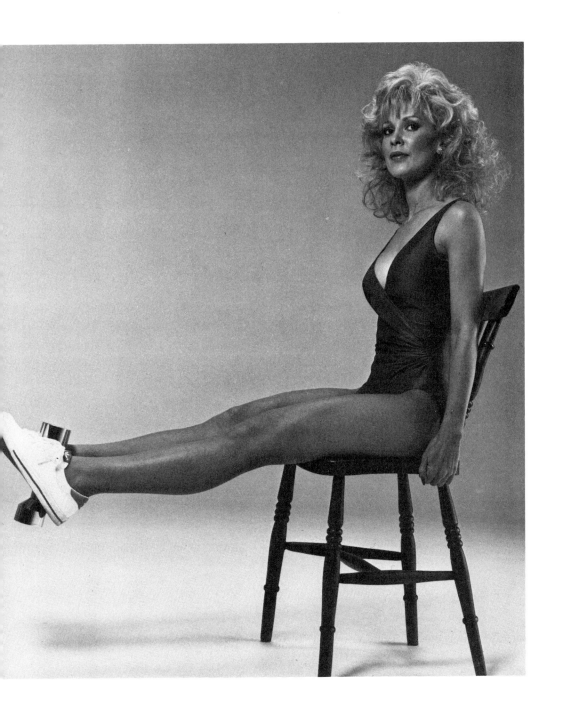

Thighs (Back and Outer)

Exercise 38: Standing Cable Leg Raises

Facing the machine, attach cable to ankle. Standing as straight as possible, extend the leg back and up. Return to starting position. Repeat all sets. This works back of the thighs. Switch legs. You can also do this exercise from the side, which works the outer thigh, or facing away from the machine, which works the front of the thigh.

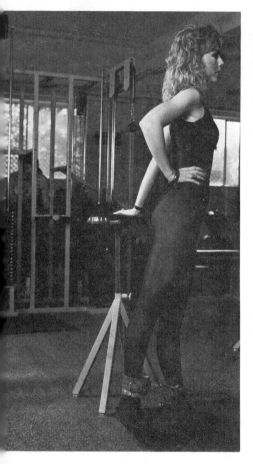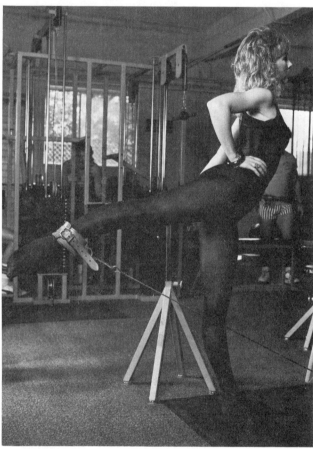

Facing machine

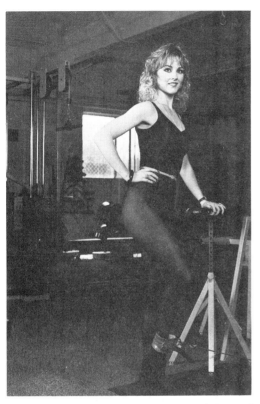
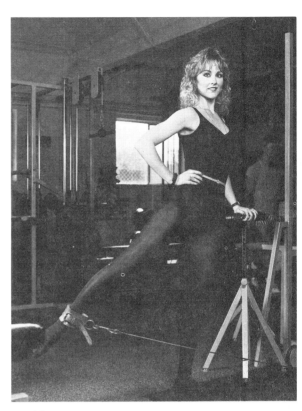

Side to the machine

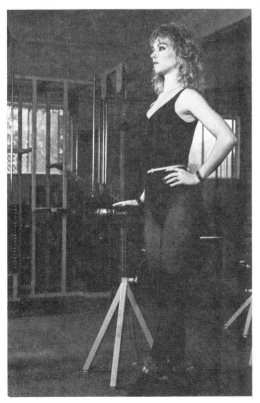
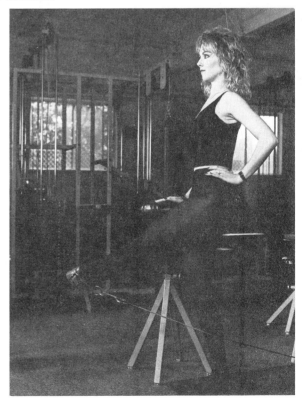

Facing away from the machine

Exercise 39: Standing Leg Raises

Stand with your feet about 10 inches apart, holding onto a chair with your left hand. Raise your right leg in front of you until your foot is at hip level. Then, in one controlled motion, move it straight back as far as it will comfortably go. Do 20 reps. Repeat with the left leg. Use 3- to 5-pound ankle weights, and you'll see quick results.

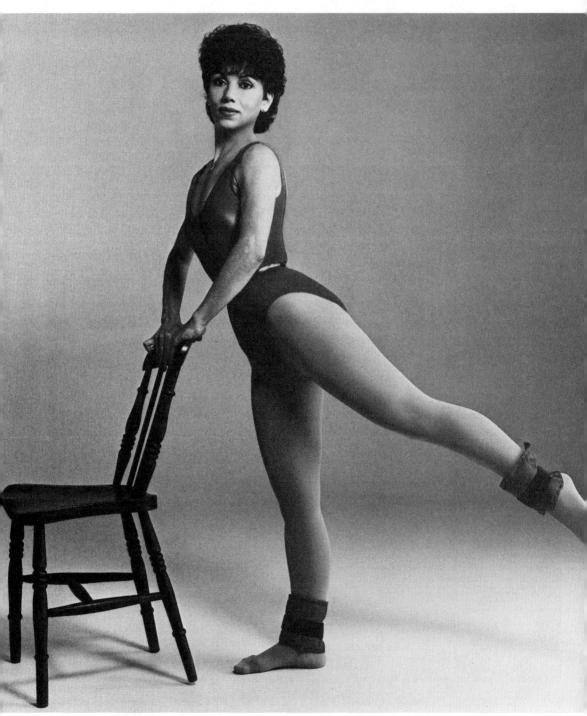

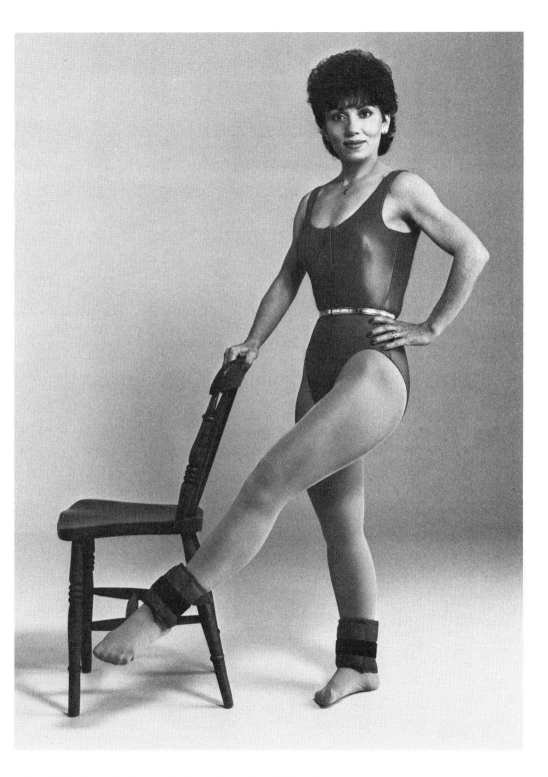

Lying Side Leg Raises with Arm Stretched Overhead
 See Exercise 5 on page 61 for description. However, use 3- to 5-pound ankle weights.

Outer Thigh Back Leg Raises
 See Exercise 8 on page 64 for description.

Exercise 40: Leg Curls

Lying on your stomach on a bench, with your hands stabilizing you as shown, hold a 5-pound weight between your feet. Bending your knees, bring your feet up until they are parallel with your hips, as shown. Lower them to the original position.

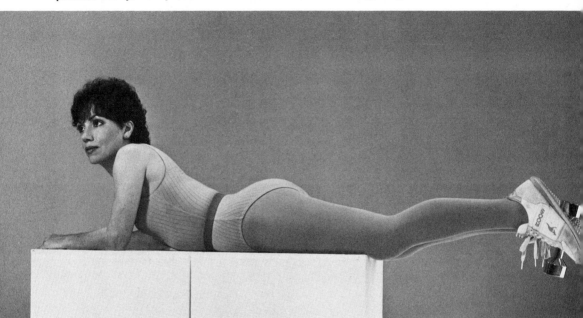

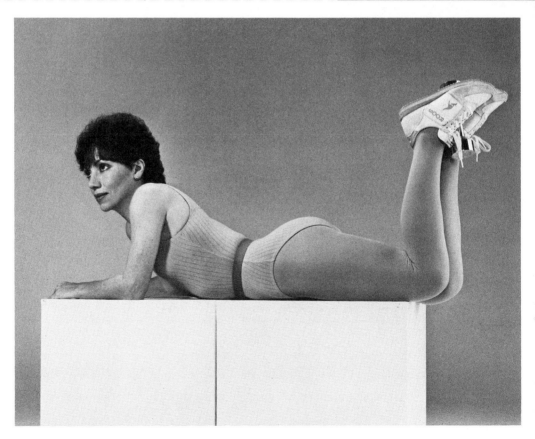

Hips

Exercise 41: Hip Lift

Kneeling on your hands and knees, fingers pointing as shown and elbows slightly bent, straighten your right leg, flexing the foot as you do so. Keeping the knee straight, raise the leg until the foot is slightly higher than the hips. Lower until the toes touch the floor. Repeat, using 3- to 5-pound weights. Do the same with the left leg.

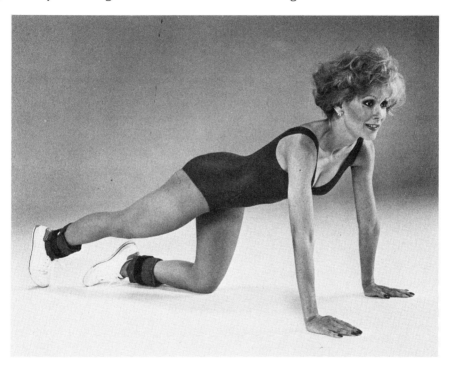

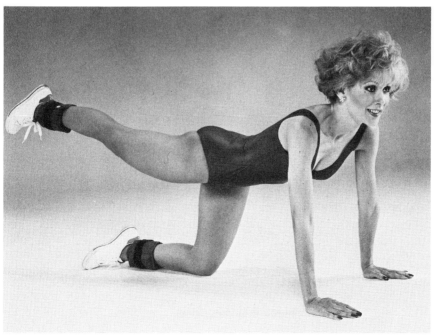

Exercise 42: Lying Hip Lift

Lie on your stomach, arms flat at your side with palms up. Toes should be resting on the floor. Flex your right foot and raise the leg as far as you can, keeping your pelvis on the floor. Lower leg. After 3 sets of 20 reps, repeat with the left leg.

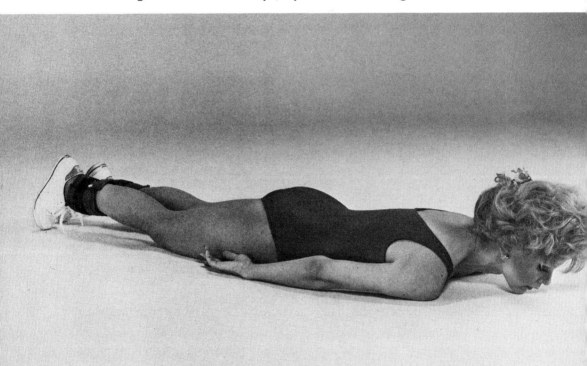

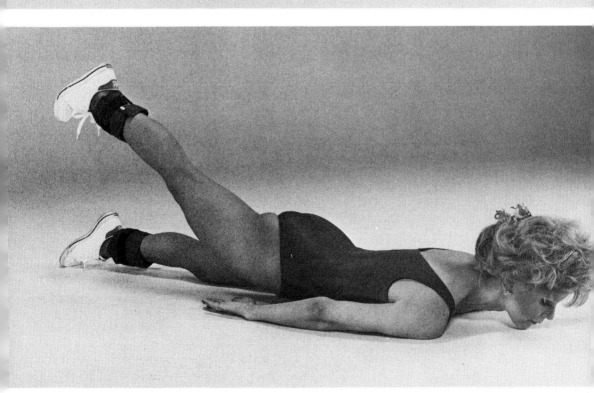

Exercise 43: Gluteus Lift

Lie on your back with your knees bent and your heels nearly touching your buttocks. Slowly lift the hips, flexing the hip muscles. Remain in this position for a few seconds before slowly lowering the hips almost to the floor. Repeat.

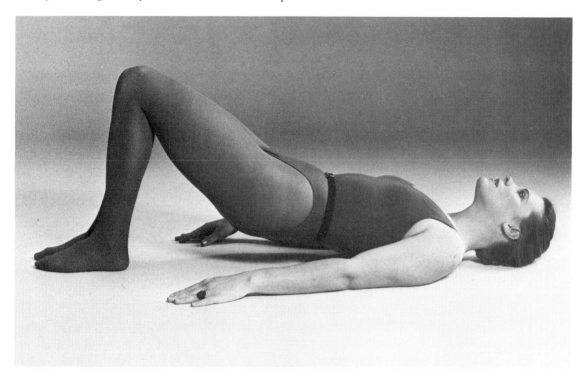

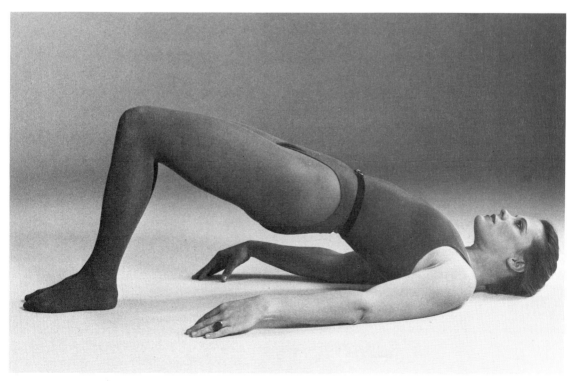

Lunges

See Exercise 13 on page 70 for description.

Squats

Dumbbell squats

See Exercise 36 on page 95 for description.

Barbell squats

See Exercise 17 on pages 74–75 for description.

Leg Curls

See Exercise 40 on page 102 for description.

Knees

Leg Extensions

See Exercise 37 on page 96 for description.

Exercise 44: Stair Climbing

One of the most effective exercises for the lower body, stair climbing can be done anywhere, even while traveling. There is no need to use weights, but try to climb at least 2 flights a day, building up to 5 each day.

> **Note:** Many people think they have naturally fat knees, when the problem is really only an accumulation of fluid owing to a sedentary lifestyle. Try using ice packs for 15 minutes, 2 times a day, for 4 weeks. Massage is also helpful, but be certain always to massage *toward* the heart. Elevate the legs at night.

Chest

To *increase* your chest dimensions, do 5 sets of 7 reps of the following exercises 3 times per week, using heavy weights. "Heavy" weights means heavy enough so that you can just complete the sets without straining. Be sure to go through a full range of motion to get the most from these exercises.

Incline Bench Press

See Exercise 14 on page 71 for description.

Incline Cross Flies

See Exercise 15 on page 72 for description.

To *reduce* your chest dimensions, do 4 sets of 20 reps of the following exercises, 6 times a week, using heavy weights.

Exercise 45: Bench Press

Begin by lifting the barbell from the stationary bench support or from your training partner. If you have neither, hold the barbell across your legs as you lie down. With the barbell supported above your chest, exhale as you straighten your arms and push up, inhale as you lower the barbell. Repeat.

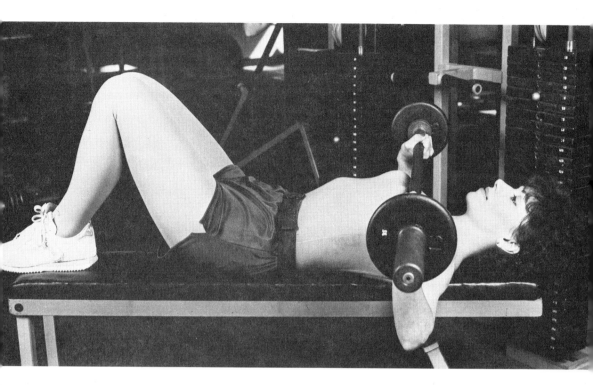

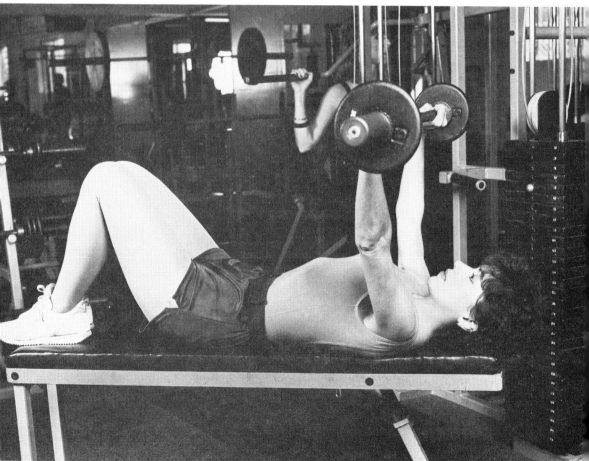

Lying Cross Flies

See Exercise 14 on page 71 for description. But do this exercise lying flat on your back.

> **Note:** Exercises such as the bench press and cross flies always reduce this area of the chest because the breast is made up of 60 percent fat and 40 percent glandular tissue, both of which tend to shrink when exercised directly. To gain, however, you must work out on a high-incline bench, doing the incline bench press and incline flies, both of which exercise the pectoralis muscles. By using heavier weights and fewer reps, the breast tissue is reduced as little as possible, while the cleavage is increased, thus making the upper breast appear larger.

Postpregnancy Tummy Flatteners

To regain your prepregnancy flat tummy, do the following program 6 times per week.

EXERCISE	SETS	REPS
Bent-Leg Sit Ups (see page 62)	1	25
Bent-Leg Raises (see page 84)	1	25
Straight-Leg Raises (see page 86)	1	25
Straight-Leg Scissors (see page 90)	1	25
Crunches (see page 88)	1	25

Repeat the program 3 times a day for the first 3 weeks, then increase exercises by 1 set every week until you are doing 6 sets of each. Continue until you have reached your goal; then do this program 3 times per week for maintenance.

7

THE ADVANCED HOME PROGRAM

This program provides a complete body workout in the convenience of your home. While some equipment is necessary, we believe you'll find that the minimal investment required will produce a maximum change in your body.

Since the intent in any program is to keep the movement and momentum going while exercising, we suggest that you arrange the weights in the order you will be using them. If you have 2 bars, you can mount the weights on the bars before you begin.

The program should be done in 2 parts, on alternating days. The first half, which primarily works the upper body, should be done 3 days per week, with the lower body workout on the alternate days.

To determine how much weight you should be lifting, practice doing the program, completing the specified number of reps for each exercise in turn. Be sure you're going through the complete range of motion required by each exercise. If the last set is difficult and you are unable to do any more, you are using the correct amount of weights. If you cannot complete the last set, you are using too much weight. If you feel able to do more after completing the last set, you should add more weight.

Equipment:
Bench that inclines
Easy curl bar
Short straight bar (4 feet long)
Long straight bar (5 to 6 feet long)
Plates for the bars in the following sizes:
    Six 2½ pounds
    Six 5 pounds
    Six 10 pounds
    Two 25 pounds
Four pairs of dumbbells:
    5 pounds
    10 pounds
    15 pounds
    25 pounds
One pair of 5-pound ankle weights
Machine for leg extensions and leg curls. This is usually found in combination with a
    bench that inclines—it's a good, multi-purpose investment.

109

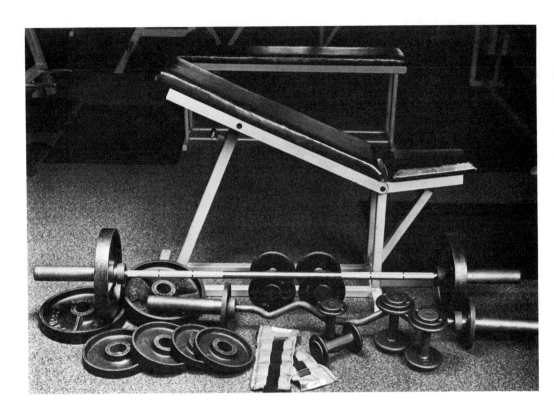

UPPER BODY PROGRAM: Day One

Warm-Up:
Stretches on pages 42–45

Exercises:
Chest:
Incline Bench Press
Incline Cross Flies

Shoulders:
Bent-Over Lateral Raises
Standing Lateral Raises
Front Raises

Back:
One-Arm Rowing
Barbell Rowing

Arms:
Lying Triceps Extension
Seated Dumbbell Curls
Bench Press Narrow Grip
Standing Barbell Curls

Stomach and Hips:
Bent-Leg Sit-Ups
Lying Side Leg Raises with Arm Stretched Overhead
Hip Lift

Incline Bench Press

See Exercise 14 on page 71 for description.
Do 4 sets of 7 reps.

Incline Cross Flies

See Exercise 15 on page 72 for description.
Do 4 sets of 7 reps.

Bent-Over Lateral Raises

See Exercise 2 on page 56 for description.
Do 4 sets of 7 reps.

Lateral Raises

See Exercise 3 on page 58 for description.
Do 4 sets of 7 reps.

Exercise 46: Front Raises

With a dumbbell in each hand, alternately raise the arms as shown. The arm raises past shoulder level, but does not lift overhead.

Do 3 sets of 7 reps.

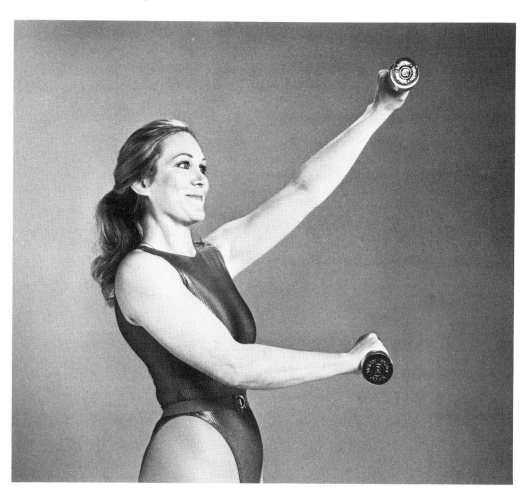

One-Arm Rowing

See Exercise 1 on page 55 for description.
Do 4 sets of 10 reps.

Barbell Rowing

See Exercise 16 on page 73 for description.
Do 4 sets of 10 reps.

Lying Triceps Extension

See Exercise 19 on page 78 for description.
Do 3 sets of 15 reps.

Seated Dumbbell Curls

See Exercise 12 on page 68 for description. In this exercise, however, sit on a bench or chair.
Do 3 sets of 7 reps.

Exercise 47: Bench Press Narrow Grip

Lie on the bench, with your hands approximately 4 to 6 inches apart, grasping the bar in an overhand grip. Inhale as you bring the bar down until your hands touch your chest, then exhale as you straighten your arms to a full extension.

Do 3 sets of 10 reps.

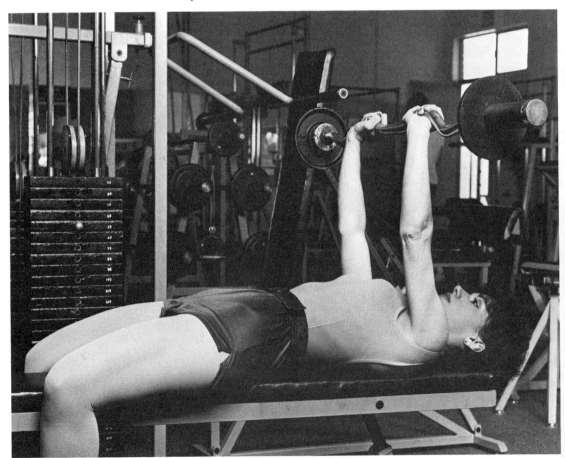

Exercise 48: *Standing Barbell Curls*

Hold the barbell in front of you, with your arms hanging straight. Using an underhand grip, curl the bar while taking care to keep the arms as close to your sides as possible.
Do 3 sets of 7 reps.

Bent-Leg Sit-Ups
See Exercise 6 on page 62 for description.
Do 3 sets of 25 reps.

Lying Side Leg Raises with Arm Stretched Overhead
See Exercise 5 on page 61 for description.
Do 3 sets of 40 reps.

Hip Lift
See Exercise 41 on page 103 for description.
Do 4 sets of 25 reps.

Warm Down:
Repeat warm-up stretches after completing program.

NOTE: This program combines triceps and biceps exercises, with more repetitions for the triceps to balance the development of the 2 upper-arm muscles. The triceps usually need to be built up.

LOWER BODY PROGRAM
(Do on alternate days)
Warm Up:
Stretches on pages 42–45

Exercises:
Thighs and legs:
Squats
Front Squats
Lunges

> *Optional:*
> Leg Extensions
> Leg Curls

Calves:
Calf Raises
Front Calf Raises

Stomach and Hips
Bent-Leg Sit-Ups
Elbow to Knee
Crunches
Lying Side Leg Raises
Lying Hip Lift
Hip Lift

NOTE: All stomach and hip exercises should be done with 5-pound ankle weights.

Squats

Dumbbell Squats:

See Exercise 36 on page 95 for description.

Barbell Squats:

See Exercise 17 on page 74 for description.

Do 3 sets of 25 reps.

Exercise 49: Front Squats

With a 3-inch block or book under your heels for balance, hold the bar across your shoulders in front of your neck as shown. Keeping your back straight, bend your knees and squat, exhaling as you bend. Inhale as you stand up.

Do 3 sets of 25 reps.

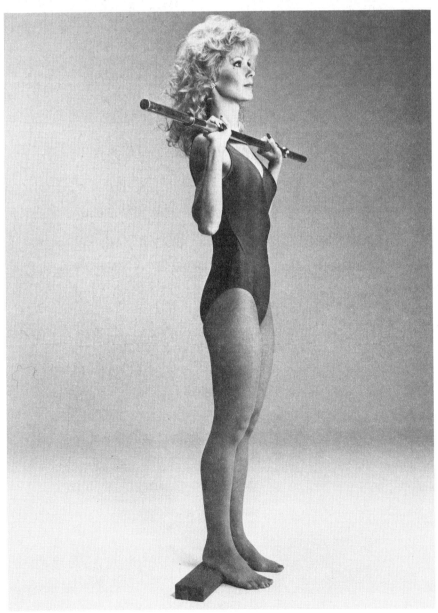

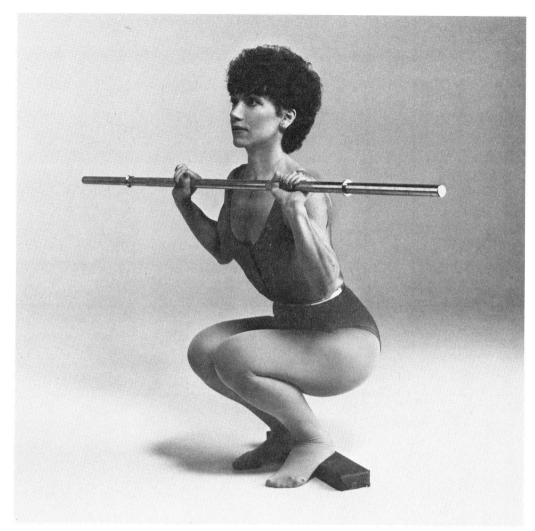

Lunges

See Exercise 13 on page 70 for description.
Do 3 sets of 25 reps.

Leg Extensions

See Exercise 37 on page 96 for description.
Do 3 sets of 20 reps.

Leg Curls

See Exercise 40 on page 102 for description.
Do 3 sets of 15 reps.

NOTE: Squats, front squats, and lunges work miracles on the hips and upper thighs, while the leg extensions work specifically on the front of the thigh. If you have a knee problem, you might find it difficult to do squats, front squats, and lunges, but leg extensions can help to strengthen the muscles surrounding the knee. In fact, the leg extension is the most commonly prescribed exercise for rehabilitation following knee injuries. Leg curls are particularly good for hamstring muscles and hips, and they can also help correct knock-knees.

Exercise 50: Calf Raises

Stand on a block of wood or on a step. Hold the back of a chair or a wall for balance. Raise up and down on the toes. You can also do the exercise on one foot at a time.

Do 5 sets of 15 reps.

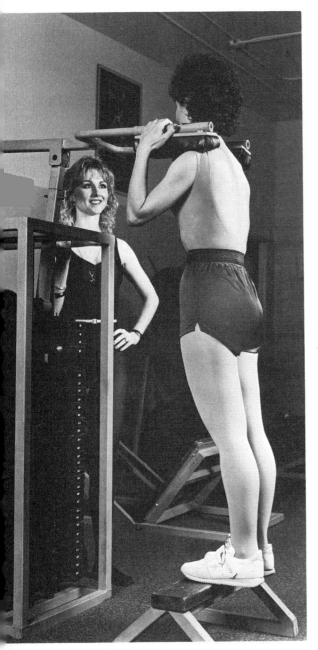 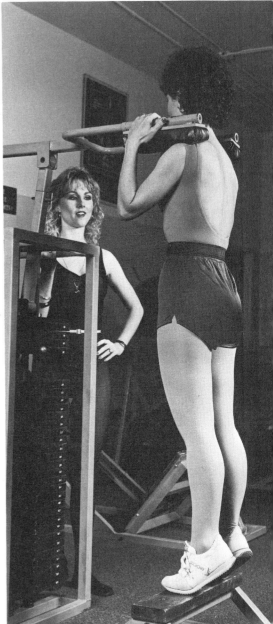

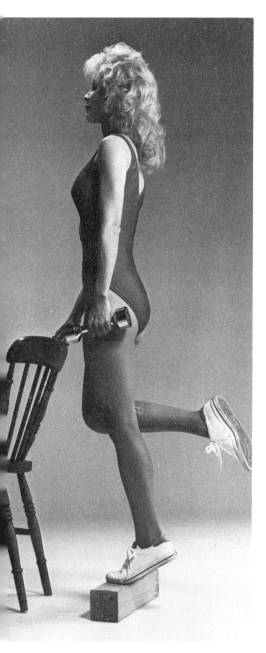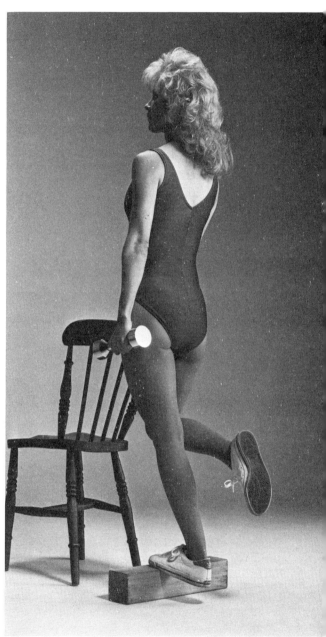

Exercise 51: Front Calf Raises

With both feet on a book or block of wood, raise up and down on heels. Lift toes, then flex down as far as possible. Use a wall or the back of a chair if necessary for balance. This exercise can also be done in a gym, as shown.

Do 5 sets of 15 reps.

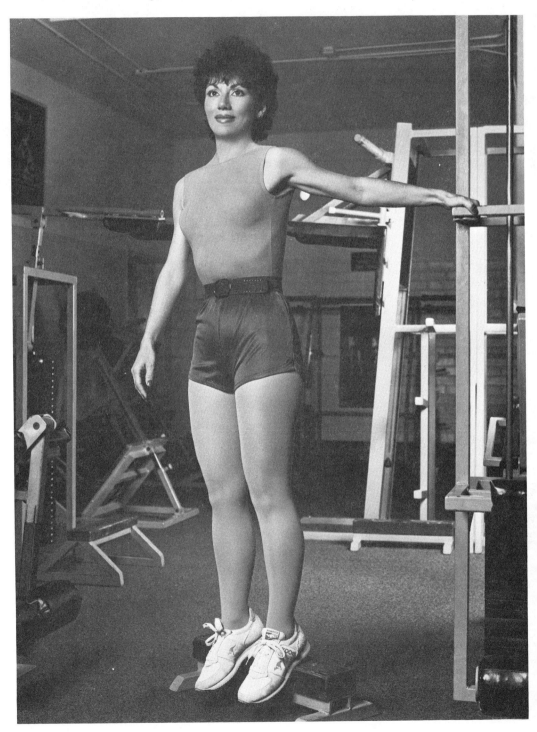

NOTE: The combination of calf raises and front calf raises is particularly good for women who wear high-heeled shoes, since the angle of those shoes tightens the back of the calf and weakens the front, causing ankle problems, shin splints, and cramps in the back of the legs. Combining these two exercises should eliminate these problems for most women.

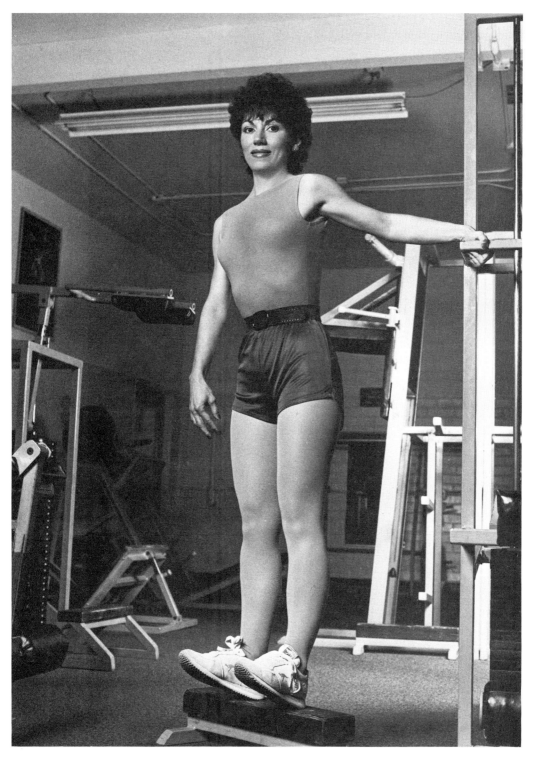

Bent-Leg Sit-Ups

See Exercise 6 on page 62 for description.
Do 3 sets of 25 reps.

Elbow to Knee

See Exercise 29 on page 87 for description.
Do 3 set of 25 reps.

Crunches

See Exercise 30 on page 88 for description.
Do 3 sets of 25 reps.

Lying Inner Thigh Leg Raises

See Exercise 34 on page 94 for description.
Do 3 sets of 25 reps.

Lying Hip Lift

See Exercise 42 on page 104 for description.
Do 3 sets of 25 reps.

Inner Thigh Back Leg Raises

See Exercise 7 on page 63 for description.
Do 3 sets of 25 reps.

Outer Thigh Back Leg Raises

See Exercise 8 on page 64 for description.
Do 3 sets of 25 reps.

8

WORKING OUT AT THE GYM

Many women ask us if there is an advantage in working out at a gym rather than doing their programs at home. Of course, gyms offer a wide variety of equipment designed to firm and trim most parts of your body. The availability of various machines makes it relatively simple to change or adapt programs to meet specific figure goals, or to accommodate your increasing strength and flexibility. Some gyms have specially designed running tracks, which reduce stress on knees and other joints. And if the gym is properly staffed by professionals, you can get expert advice to make certain you are doing the exercises properly. Many women also find it more challenging to exercise in a gym, since they push themselves a bit harder in a competitive environment.

There are other advantages as well. It's a real luxury to be able to finish off your workout with a dip in the pool, or to pamper yourself with a few minutes in the steam room or jacuzzi. And particularly posh gyms even have hair-styling and manicure facilities.

But the real reason you join a gym is to exercise, and we cannot deny that paying for a gym membership has a way of making most women more diligent in following their workout programs.

So it's up to you. If you can afford to go to a gym, fine. But remember that the crowds at many facilities may make it necessary for you to wait 10 minutes or more to use the more popular machines, thus interrupting your momentum. If you do have access to a gym, try to plan your sessions for off-peak times so that you can progress through your workout with as little delay as possible between exercises.

This chapter offers three programs that utilize the equipment available at most gyms. Included are a Beginner's Three-Day-a-Week Program, an Intermediate/Advanced/Maintenance Three-Day-a-Week Program, and a Super Results Six-Day-a-Week Program designed to take your body to its maximum peak of performance and fitness. The last program can be used for women's body-building training, as our makeover model, Suzette, is doing.

All of the programs are grouped together, followed by a glossary of the recommended exercises. We've repeated the descriptions of exercises that are also done in the home programs, so that the complete at-the-gym guide is conveniently contained in this one chapter.

BEGINNER'S THREE-DAY-A-WEEK PROGRAM

This program is ideal for the woman who is just beginning to work out in a gym. It combines a thorough all-over firming and toning workout while increasing strength, stamina, and flexibility.

As with the free-weight-training programs, we recommend that you do the exercises in the sequence in which they are given. Doing exercises in sequence takes advantage of the increased blood flow to specific areas of the body, maximizing the effectiveness of each exercise. And, although some people recommend doing stomach exercises at the beginning of each session, we have placed those activities at the end because, at that point, the entire body is heated up and sweating, which helps burn off abdominal fat more quickly.

EXERCISES	SETS	REPS
Incline Bench Press	3	7
Lateral Raises	3	12
Pulldowns	3	15
Triceps Pushdowns	3	15
Seated Dumbbell Curls	2	10
Leg Extensions	2	20
Leg Curl	2	15
Squats	2	15
Calf Raises	2	15
Front Calf Raises	2	15
Bent-Leg Sit-Ups	3	20
Lying Side Leg Raises with		
Arm Stretched Overhead	3	25
Inner Thigh Back Leg Raises	3	25
Outer Thigh Back Leg Raises	3	25

INTERMEDIATE/ADVANCED/MAINTENANCE THREE-DAY-A-WEEK PROGRAM

EXERCISE	SETS	REPS
Incline Bench Press	3	7
Incline Cross Flies	2	7
Lateral Raises	3	7
Seated Press	3	10
Pulldowns	4	20
Pulley Rowing	2	10

EXERCISE	SETS	REPS
Triceps Pushdowns	4	15
Seated Dumbbell Curls	3	8
Squat	2	20
Leg Curls	2	25
Calf Raises	3	15
Front Calf Raises	3	15
Bent Leg Sit-Ups	3	25
Lying Side Leg Raises with Arm Stretched Overhead	3	50

SUPER RESULTS SIX-DAY-A-WEEK SPLIT PROGRAM

Like the Advanced Home Program, this program is divided into 2 parts to be done on alternating days. This first portion exercises the upper body and stomach and should be done 3 days per week, with the lower body portion to be done on alternate days.

DAY ONE: *CHEST, BACK, SHOULDERS, ARMS & STOMACH— 3 TIMES PER WEEK*

EXERCISE	SETS	REPS
Incline Bench Press	4	7
Incline Flies	3	7
Pulldowns	4	15
Barbell Rowing	2	15
Pulley Rowing	2	15
Bent-Over Lateral Raises	3	10
Lateral Raises	3	10
Front Raises	2	10
Triceps Pushdowns	4	12
Seated Dumbbell Curls	3	8
Bench Press (Narrow Grip)	3	12
Preacher's Curls	3	8
Crunches	3	25
Lying Side Leg Raises with Arm Stretched Overhead	3	40
Donkey Kicks	3	40

DAY TWO: *HIPS, THIGHS, CALVES, STOMACH—3 TIMES PER WEEK*

EXERCISE	SETS	REPS
Calf Raises	4	15
Donkey Raises	4	15
Front Calf Raises	4	15
Leg Extension	4	25
Leg Curls	3	25
Squat	2	20
Front Squat	2	20
Bent-Leg Sit-Ups	3	30
Lying Side Leg Raises		
With Arm Stretched Overhead	3	50
Inner Thigh Back Leg Raises	3	40
Outer Thigh Back Leg Raises	3	40

GLOSSARY OF AT-THE-GYM EXERCISES

Exercise 52: Inner Thigh Back Leg Raises

On your hands and knees, as shown on page 63, extend your right leg, flex your right foot, and point your toes in, toward your other leg. Raise your leg as high as possible while keeping it tensed. Lower your leg, and repeat.

Exercise 53: Outer Thigh Back Leg Raises

On your hands and knees, as shown on page 64, extend your right leg, flex your right foot, and point your toes out, away from your other leg. Raise your leg as high as possible while keeping it tensed. Lower your leg, and repeat.

Exercise 54: Barbell Rowing

Bending forward at the waist, grasp the barbell with palms down as shown on page 73. Lift bar to chest and lower. Repeat.

Exercise 55: Bench Press

Lie down on bench and, keeping spine aligned, lift the barbell until arms are straight as shown on page 112. Lower to chest, and repeat.

Exercise 56: Bent-Leg Sit-Ups

Lie on back with legs straight and hands stretched overhead. Bend knees to chest as you bring arms forward, toward knees, raising shoulders only slightly off the ground as shown on page 62. Keep spine flat on the floor.

Exercise 57: Bent-Over Lateral Raises

Stand with feet shoulder-width apart and knees bent slightly. With elbows bent, hold dumbbells in each hand, bend forward from the waist and lift the weights to the side as shown on pages 56–57.

Exercise 58: Seated Press

Sitting straight facing the seated press machine, hold the handle with an overhand grip. Push the bar up until the arms are straight. Slowly pull down to chest level. (See pages 126–27.)

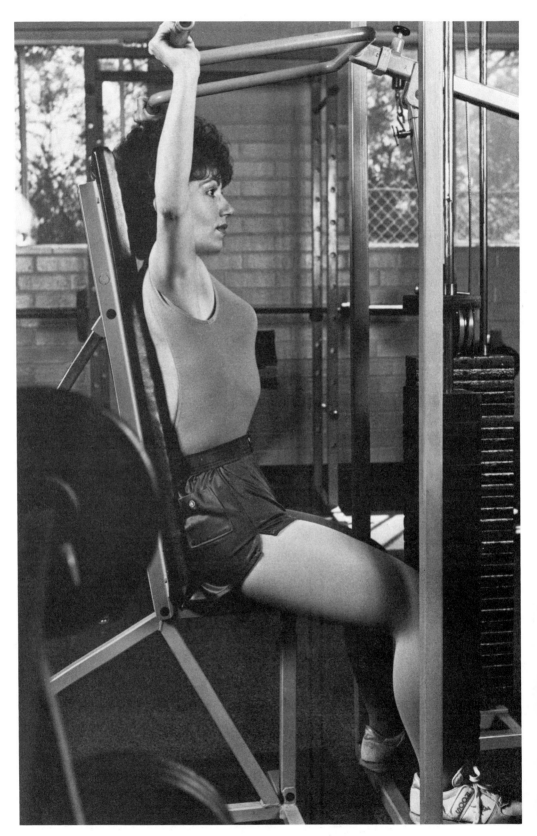

Seated press

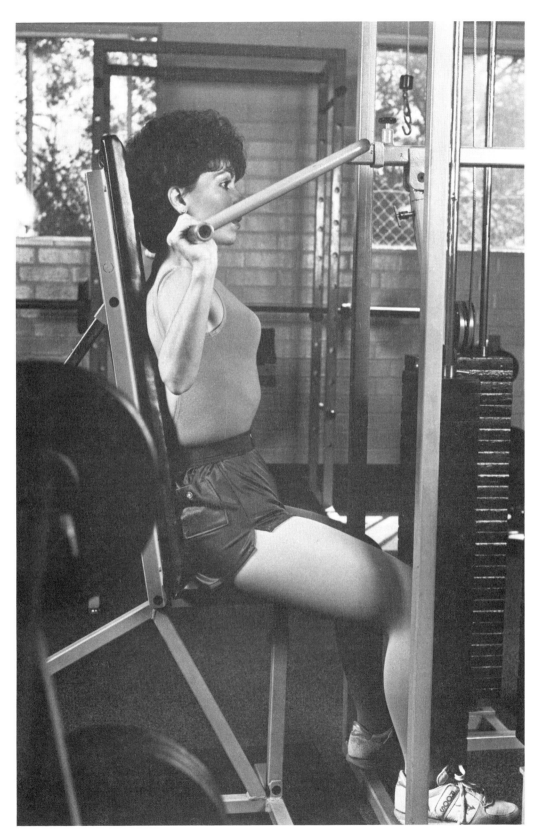

Seated press

Exercise 59: Incline Cross Flies

Sit back on the incline bench, holding a dumbbell in each hand. With arms extended toward the floor as shown on page 72, raise both arms straight up and cross them over your chest. Keep the movements smooth and controlled.

Exercise 60: Crunches

Lie on the floor with knees bent and calves supported on the seat of a chair as shown on pages 88–89. Clasp your hands over your chest and raise your upper body toward your knees.

Exercise 61: Donkey Kicks

Positioned on hands and knees with spine straight and pelvis slightly tilted, bring right knee to chest and then extend it back straight and up, keeping the buttocks and thigh muscles tight at all times.

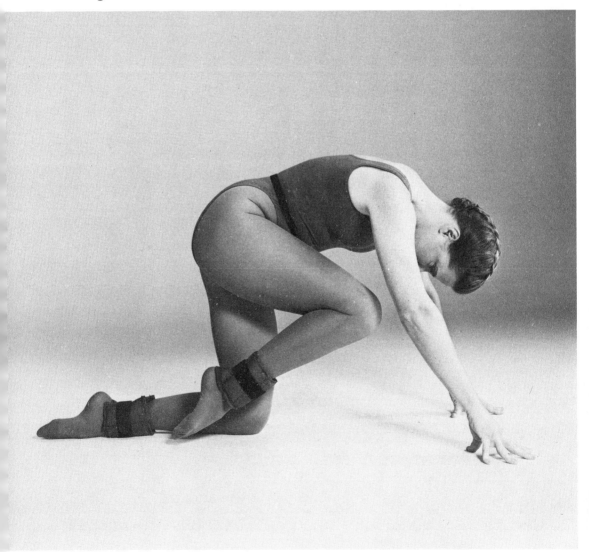

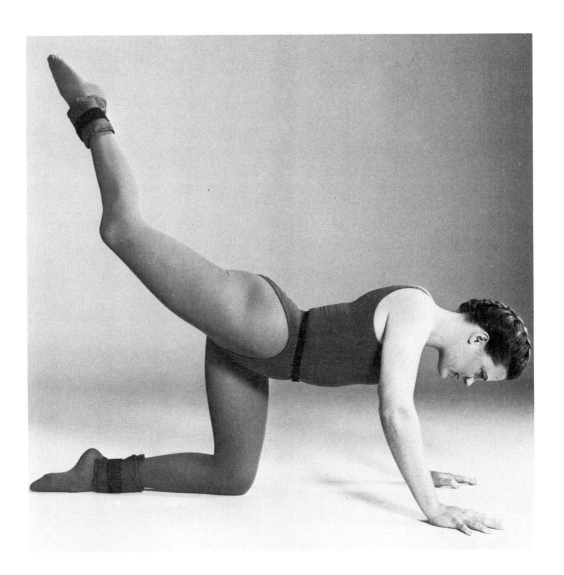

Exercise 62: Donkey Raises

This is an advanced exercise for the calves and is more effective than simple calf raises. Your training partner sits on your back, as illustrated, while you bend forward on your toes and raise and lower your heels. (See pages 130–31.)

129

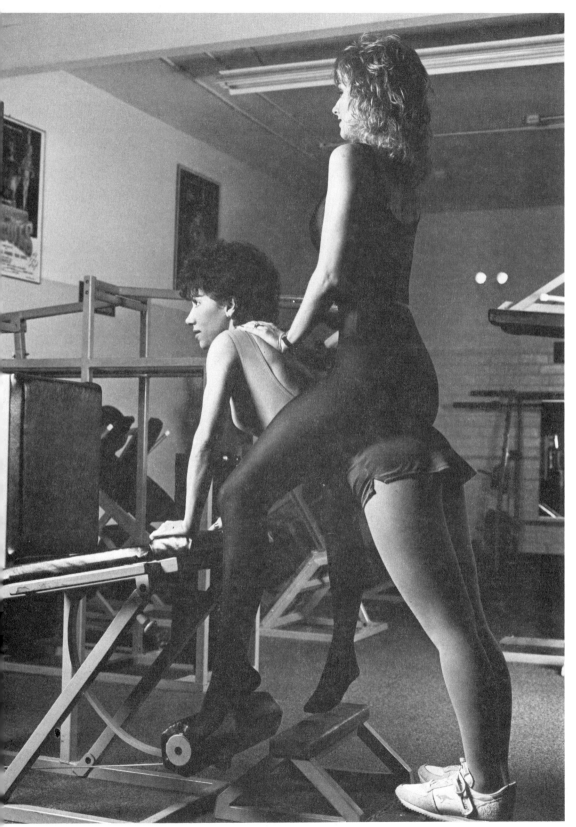

Donkey raises

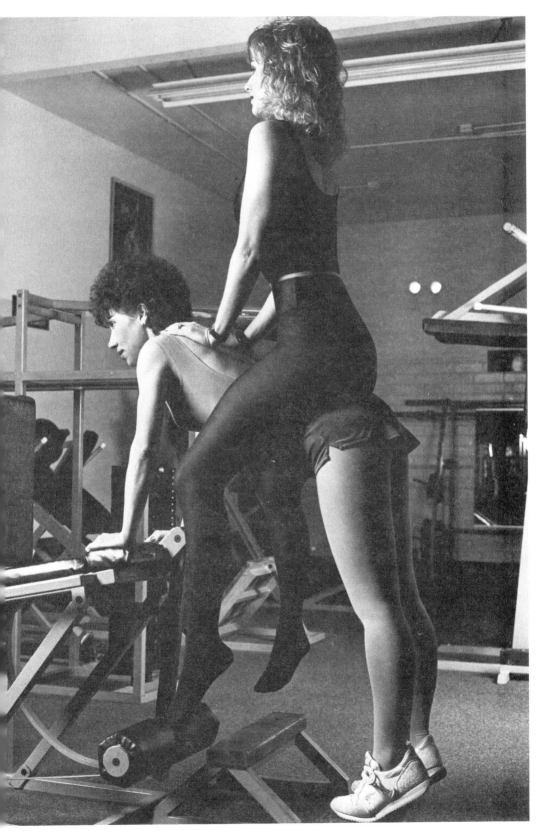

Donkey raises

Exercise 63: Incline Flies

Sit back on an incline bench. With arms slightly bent, grasp the dumbbells and hold them out at your sides, as shown. Raise the weights until they almost meet over your chest. Return to starting position.

Exercise 64: Front Calf Raises

With both feet on a book or block of wood, rise up and down on heels. Lift toes, then flex down as far as possible. Use a wall or the back of a chair if necessary for balance. See pages 118–19 for photos.

Exercise 65: Front Squats

Use a book or block of wood under your heels for proper balance. Hold a bar or bar with weights in front of your neck. Keeping your back straight, squat as low as you can. Keep the movement smooth, and don't aim for speed until you can maintain a straight back. (See photos, pages 114–15.)

Exercise 66: Barbell Bench Press

Lie on a bench with back straight. Lift the barbell until your arms are straight. Lower it to your shoulders. Exhale as you push it back up to the starting position.

Exercise 67: Dumbbell Bench Press

This exercise is done exactly the same way as the preceding Barbell Bench Press, except that this time you hold dumbbells.

Exercise 68: Lateral Raises

With feet shoulder-width apart and body slightly bent from the waist, hold dumbbells down in front of you. Keeping elbows straight, raise arms to the side until dumbbells are slightly higher than shoulder level, as shown on pages 58–59. Return to starting position.

Exercise 69: Leg Curls

Lie on your stomach on a bench, with hands holding the front grips of the bench for support as shown. Slightly raise your chest off the bench as you bend your legs at the knees, pulling the resistance mechanism toward your buttocks. Keep the movement rapid and smooth.

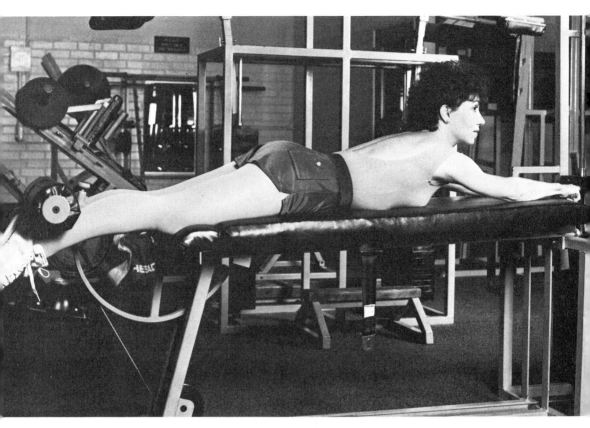

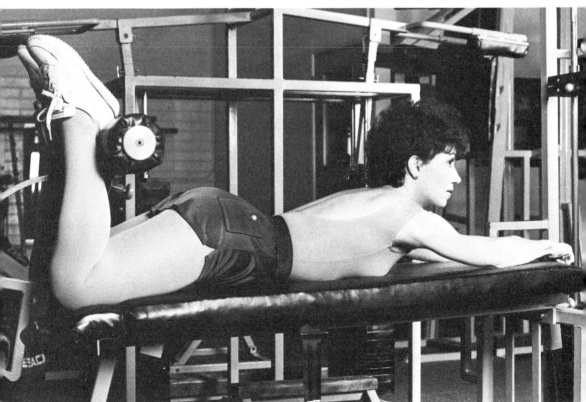

133

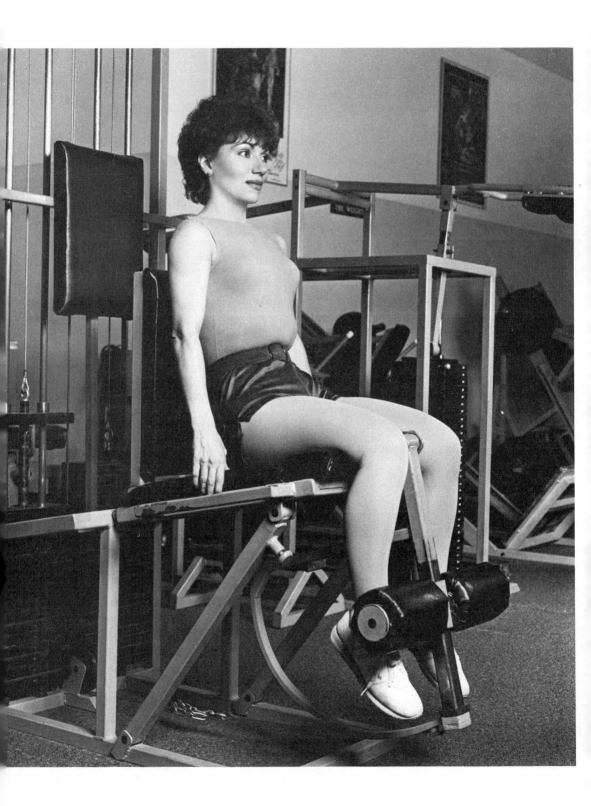

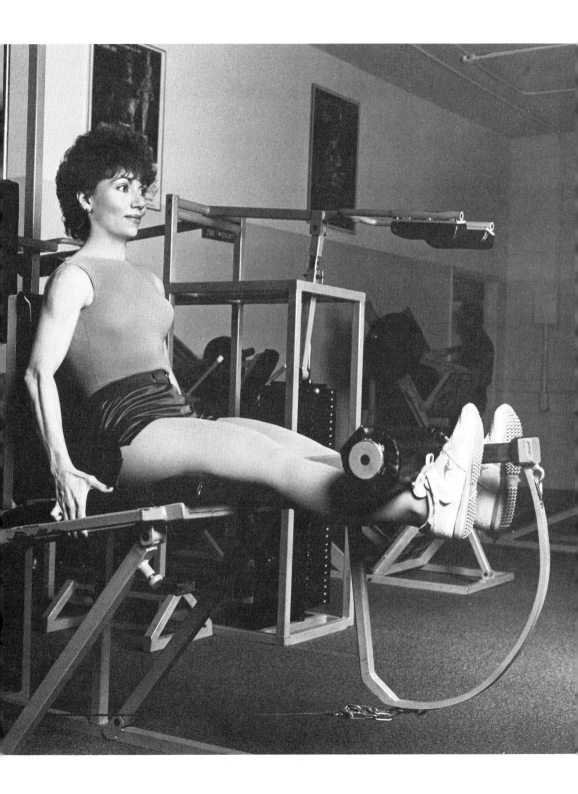

Exercise 71: Lying Side Leg Raises with Arm Stretched Overhead

Lie on right side with right leg bent at knee and left leg outstretched. Use right arm for support, and stretch left hand overhead, as shown on page 61. Lift arm to meet leg. Return to starting position, making sure to stretch both arm and leg. Repeat rapidly. Then switch to the other side.

Exercise 72: Preacher's Curls

Lean over a curling bench (or if you're doing this at home, pad the back of a chair with a pillow) as shown, and curl the barbell up toward your chin. Lower. Repeat the movement smoothly. Hands should be about 10 to 14 inches apart, and elbows must be positioned directly under your hands.

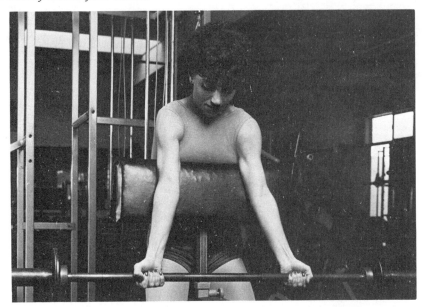

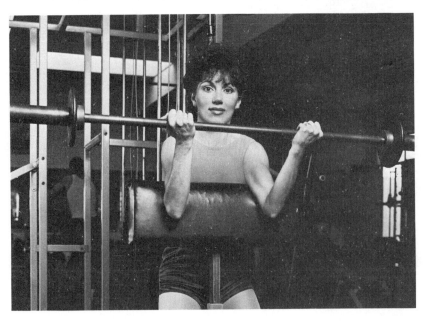

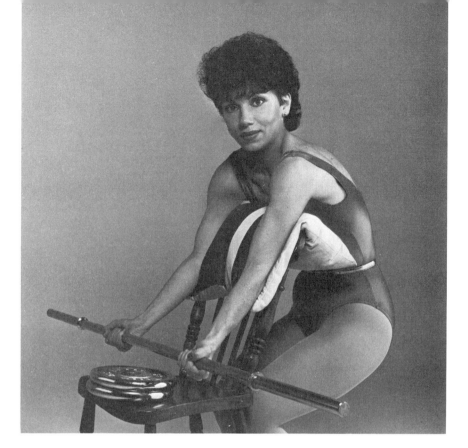

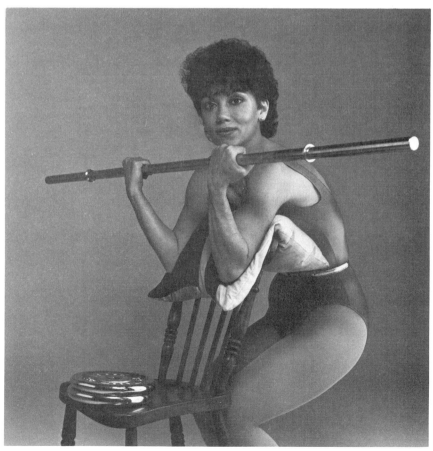

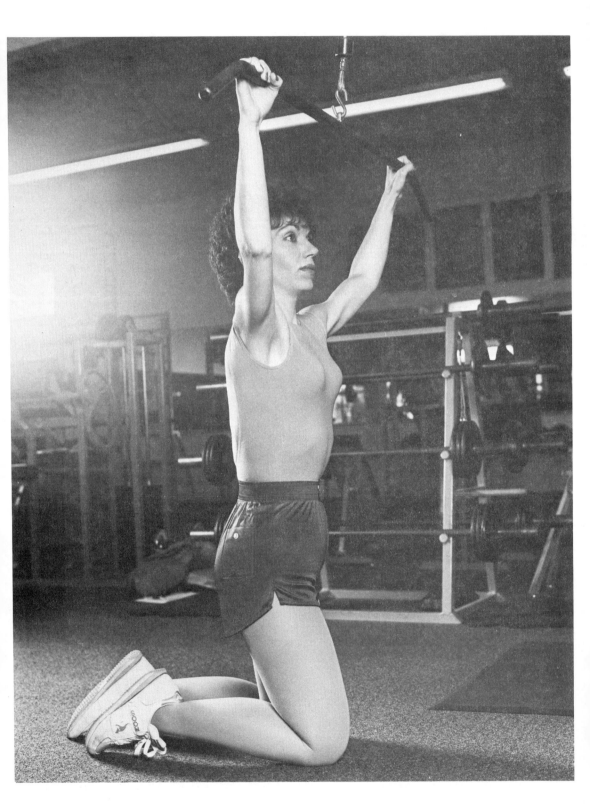

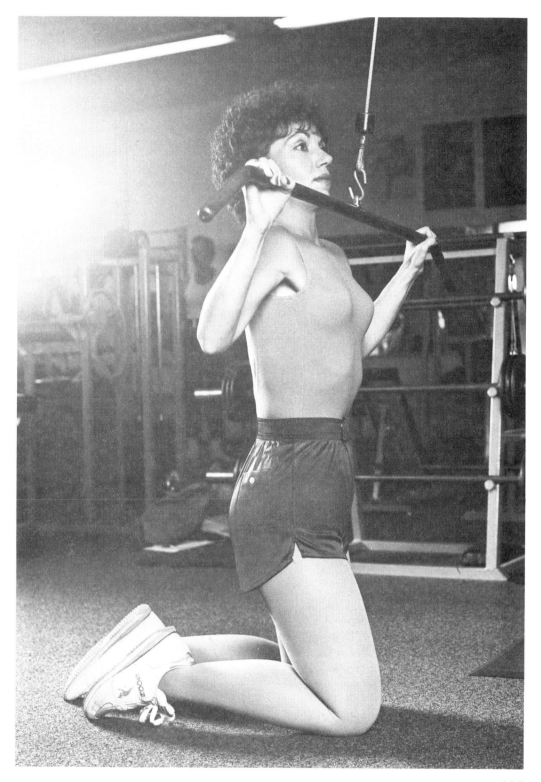

Exercise 74: Pulley Rowing

Sit facing the pulleys with legs outstretched and grab the pulley handles. Pull the handles toward your chest, bending your elbows. Using a rowing motion, bend forward as the pulleys return to the starting position.

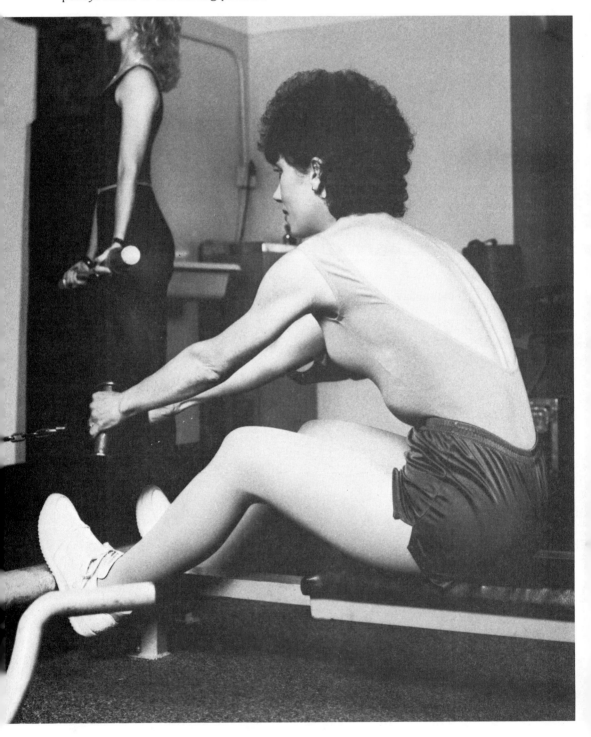

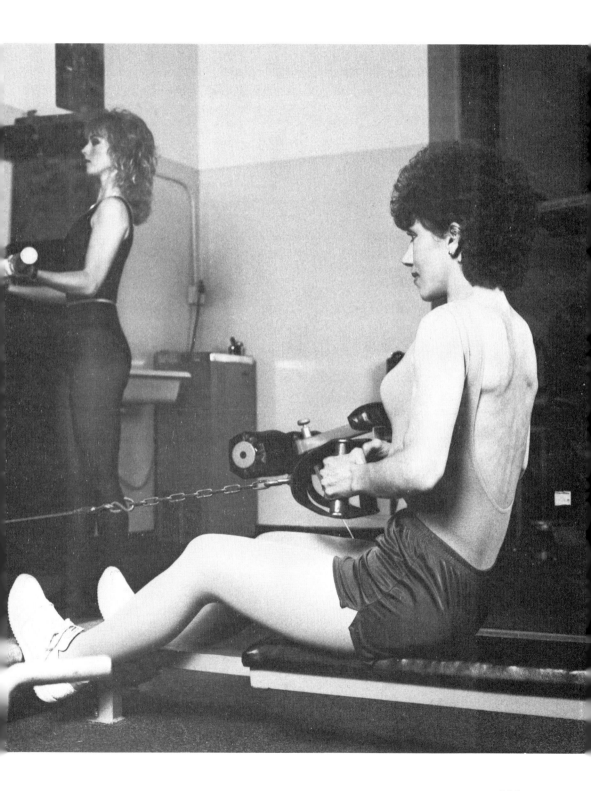

Exercise 75: Seated Dumbbell Curls

With 10-pound dumbbells in each hand, sit on a chair or bench with your arms at your sides, palms facing in. Inhale as you bring the dumbbells up, turning the hands as you do so, as shown on pages 68–69. Exhale as you bring arms down to the original position.

Exercise 76: Barbell Squats

Stand straight with a book or block of wood under your heels. With a bar across the shoulders as shown on pages 74–75, bend the knees and squat. Keeping back straight and maintaining balance, stand up. Repeat.

Exercise 77: Calf Raises

Stand on a block of wood or on a step. Hold the back of a chair or a wall for balance. Raise up and down on the toes as shown on pages 116–17. You can also do the exercise on one foot at a time.

Exercise 78: Triceps Pushdowns

Hold the bar with both hands and push down until arms are straight as shown on pages 76–77. Exhale as you push. Repeat rapidly and smoothly.

9

OVERTRAINING AND STRESS

We all know people who begin fitness programs because they want to look and feel better, but then allow that healthy goal to turn into an obsession. Little by little, they lose interest in everything except how many miles they ran that morning and how many reps they did with the barbell the night before. They lose the attractive appearance of physical fitness and develop a gaunt, tired look. They start to catch colds more frequently, and complain of being accident-prone. Shin splints, stress fractures, sprains, and strains start to occur with greater frequency. But they try to ignore these injuries, and rarely miss a day of training. They don't realize that, instead of being well-rounded individuals with enthusiasm for all that life offers, they have become boring, their one-track minds focused solely on fitness, exercise, and diet. And worst of all, they are now harming, rather than helping, their bodies.

It's true that your body thrives on activity and deteriorates if you don't move it. In fact, the physical functions upon which your health depends—circulation, oxygenation, digestion, elimination—all work best in a body that's primed by exercise and activity. Exercise increases the flow of blood to the brain, enhancing reasoning and memory function. It improves the texture and appearance of your skin, since new blood is always replenishing it. For the same reason, your hair shines, and you glow all over.

Some people, however, fall into the trap of overtraining or overexercising. They reason that if a moderate amount is good, then a lot must be better, right? Wrong! An over-trained body is just like any other piece of machinery that has been pushed beyond its limit; it is more likely to break down, since it's operating under constant stress. Continued fatigue and frequent colds and flu attacks are signs that your body's immune system is being over-worked and therefore is not functioning properly. Good health is the result of *balance* in our lives—balance between work and rest, activity and leisure.

We've said that proper exercise and a suitable weight-training program will improve your body and your life. But we don't want you to exchange a sedentary life for one as a compulsive athlete. Exercise should become an important part of your life, but that's all it should be—*part* of your life. Just as you shouldn't let your job or your family or a new romance consume your every waking moment, you should also remember to keep exercise and weight training in their proper perspective.

Your body is a miraculous machine, and it instinctively tries to maintain homeostasis or balance. Listen to it. It will tell you when to slow down and, believe us, it knows best.

OVERTRAINING: THE WARNING SIGNALS

Be alert for the symptoms of overtraining. Heed their warning, or you'll do your body more harm than good. When you suspect that any of these symptoms are caused by overtraining, take a week or two off from your training program. Substitute a brisk 45-minute walk 3 to 4 times a week. After your break, gradually get back into your training routine.

1. CONSTANT FATIGUE

It's normal to feel tired after a good workout or at the end of a busy day. But if you find yourself always responding to the question, "How are you?" with, "Tired," then consider the possibility that you may be overtraining.

2. INSOMNIA

A properly balanced exercise program should contribute to sound, healthful sleep. If you find yourself repeatedly tossing and turning at night, you're probably overtraining. If you've been working out at night, try switching to a morning schedule.

3. INJURIES

Most injuries occur when people have pushed their bodies beyond a reasonable limit. Don't ask your body to do more than it was meant to, or you'll pay a price in sprains, strains, or worse.

4. LOSS OF APPETITE

While exercise will help you to control your appetite, excessive exercise can cause loss of appetite, resulting in poor nutrition and greater vulnerability to illness and injuries. If you find yourself skipping meals because you simply aren't hungry, realize that this could be a warning.

5. INCREASED PULSE RATE

Sports, exercise, and weight training are beneficial in improving cardio-vascular conditioning because they temporarily speed up the pulse, thus bringing more oxygen to the muscles and organs of the body. But that increased rate is only temporary. A balanced exercise program results in a resting pulse that is average or below average for your age, height, and weight. A constantly elevated pulse rate is a warning that your heart is working harder than it should. Rest several days until your pulse returns to normal.

To find your resting pulse rate, take your pulse immediately upon waking in the morning. Count the beat for 15 seconds, then multiply by 4. The average is 72. When you exercise vigorously, your pulse should never exceed your own maximum heart rate. Calculate your MHR by subtracting your age from 220 (the maximum number of beats per minute possible for the average heart), then multiply by .70 (you should work at no more than 70 percent of your maximum heart rate). A 35-year-old woman should train so that her pulse is no more than 136–137 $(220 - 35 = 185 \times .70 = 136.5)$. To take your working pulse during exercise, count for only 6 seconds and then multiply by 10. The reason for this is that the pulse slows very rapidly upon cessation of exercise. A 15-second count is often misleading.

6. MUSCLE WEAKNESS

When muscles are overworked, they grow weaker rather than stronger and are much more susceptible to injury. Your muscles need at least 48 hours to recover after heavy weight training, which is why we advocate split routines in the advanced programs. You exercise upper body muscles one day, the lower body the next. Repeated minor sprains and strains are a clear sign of overtraining.

7. MUSCLE SORENESS

It's normal to be sore for a few days after beginning a weight-training program and after each increase in reps, sets, or weights. It's also normal to feel a slight soreness after a good workout. But if your muscles stay sore for more than 5 days, you could be training too rigorously. Increase your intake of Vitamin C and rest for a week. Then begin training again, but less intensively.

8. LOWERED RESISTANCE

Just about everyone is susceptible to colds and the flu from time to time, but if you start to have frequent colds or catch every flu bug that comes around, you may need to cut down on your training schedule. Pay particular attention to your diet and nutritional supplements.

9. BODY STOPS RESPONDING TO EXERCISE

Your body will soon show you when you're overtraining. For example, when you stop improving in strength and tone, it's an indication that training is no longer building up, but breaking down your body, by weakening your muscles. Stop training for 1 to 2 weeks. Then gradually work back into a sensible training schedule.

10. GENERAL WEAKNESS

General weakness and malaise may be an indication that your body is being depleted of essential vitamins and minerals, a common side effect of overtraining. Rest for 1 to 2 weeks and take vitamin and mineral supplements (see Chapter 13 on nutrition).

HOOKED ON EXERCISE?

Some researchers suggest that exercise can actually become physically addicting, owing to the morphine-like hormone, beta-endorphin, which is secreted by the brain after prolonged exercise. This substance produces a stimulating, pleasurable "high," while reducing depression and anxiety. A certain amount of this hormone is beneficial and can make life in this stress-filled world a lot easier. But overtraining can actually result in a craving for beta-endorphin which can only be satisifed by more and more exercise. As with all addictions, the best answer is simply to avoid becoming "hooked." Exercise should be a pleasant, healthful part of your life, but that's all it should be.

AMENORRHEA

While a balanced program of exercise and good nutrition generally results in better health and stamina, too much exercise can produce an unexpected side effect—amenorrhea, or irregular menstrual periods. Studies of women athletes indicate that as many as half of all women participating in strenuous exercise experience changes in their menstrual pattern. These changes are particularly pronounced when there is a dramatic drop in the percentage of body fat. Some experts say that menstrual irregularities are likely to occur whenever body fat drops below 8–12 percent, while for other researchers the threshold is lower. Thaddeus Kostrubala, M.D., co-author of *The Joy of Running*, says that strenuous athletic conditioning actually causes changes in the hypothalamus, the part of the brain that serves as a regulatory and controlling center. He warns that it is sometimes difficult for an interrupted menstrual cycle to return to normal, and that the difficulty is increased the longer the cycle has been stopped.

Other studies have shown that young women whose periods are interrupted by strenuous physical activity are extremely vulnerable to the bone-weakening condition called osteoporosis. Brittle bones have usually been associated with older women, whose estrogen levels are greatly reduced after menopause. Estrogen, the female sex hormone, serves to protect the bones. But, with the increased numbers of women who are overtraining to the point of stopping their menstrual periods, the number of cases of osteoporosis even in women in their 20s, 30s, and 40s has grown.

If your periods stop from over-exercise and dieting, it's a sign that your body is not working properly. Never exercise so intensely that your body stops functioning properly and your hormones get out of balance. Fat is needed for insulation, protection of the organs, and proper hormonal functions. Overtime hormonal imbalances can drastically affect your body's natural immune system and make you more susceptible to illness. If there is one message we hope you get from this book, it is the importance of *balance*. A body that has ceased menstruating is no longer in proper balance. Listen to your body, reduce your training schedule, and modify your diet to regain needed body fat. You'll be healthier, happier, and more attractive.

A NOTE ABOUT P.M.S.

While overtraining can result in amenorrhea, moderate training has been shown to be extremely effective for alleviating the depression, cramping, bloating, and other symptoms associated with premenstrual syndrome (P.M.S.). These symptoms usually occur anywhere from 2 to 14 days before the onset of the menstrual period, so weight training during this time is very important. Increased intake of vitamins and minerals as soon as P.M.S. symptoms occur may also be helpful.

We suggest an increase of Vitamin B-6 to 500–600 mg/day; 400 units of Vitamin D 3 times a day; 80 to 120 milli-equivalents (mEq.) of potassium; 300 mg of iron 3 times a day (daily, not just during the P.M.S. period); 30 mg of zinc daily, increasing to 50 mg during the premenstrual period; for severe cramping, 500 mg of calcium gluconate with 250 mg magnesium every hour until cramping subsides. Excess calcium is usually eliminated from the body naturally, but women who have a condition that requires attention to calcium levels in the body should consult a health-care professional.

Unless your body tells you to, there is no reason to reduce your training program during the P.M.S. period. During the menstrual cycle, training may help to relieve the cramping sensations. However, overtraining during these critical weeks can cause a hormonal imbalance and physical exertion, both of which will exaggerate the P.M.S. symptoms.

NO PAIN, NO GAIN?

We do not believe in the slogan, "No pain, no gain." In fact, pain is a clear indication that something is wrong, either with the exercise you are doing or the way you are doing it. It is normal to feel some soreness after your muscles have worked hard, but actual pain either during or after a workout is a warning. Check to make certain that you are doing the exercise correctly. If you are still experiencing pain, try lifting lighter weights. If there is still pain, perform in turn each exercise in your workout that involves the area that is in pain; you should be able to isolate the one that is causing the problem. At that point, check your form again to see if you're doing the exercise correctly. If you are, and you continue to experience pain, eliminate that exercise from your program. Body structures vary, and not all exercises are good for everyone. Once again, listen to your body.

A NOTE ABOUT DRUGS

Even the most innocent-sounding drugs can affect your performance. Don't be surprised if when you take aspirin, you find that you are sore after a training period. Aspirin masks the slight pains during a workout that are your normal signals to slow down. Those antihistamine pills that you take for colds and flu can cause drowsiness and affect your coordination, so don't take them if you're working out—or vice versa. The levels of caffeine in your system after drinking too much coffee, tea, and cola drinks can also disturb your precision of movement, and could result in injuries. Alcohol has the same effect, only worse! But take heart; the more you exercise and improve your health and stamina, the less you'll need of any of these drugs.

STRESS

From time to time, women who have been achieving good results with their program suddenly find themselves at a plateau. They stop losing weight; they may even put a few pounds back on. Their training becomes difficult and labored, and their energy level falters. Unfortunately, they sometimes conclude that their program has stopped working for them. "What's the use," they shrug, and abandon all the good habits they've struggled so hard to acquire.

The culprit is usually stress, the common companion for many of us in our busy lives. Stress can create tremendous problems for the woman who is serious about redesigning her body, because in periods of high stress:

- The body doesn't digest food as well, thus making it more difficult to diet and lose weight.

- Because elimination is slowed down, the body retains more fluid, which may even cause a temporary weight gain.

- The body doesn't respond as usual to exercise, because stress is tiring and drains energy.

- Both stress and fatigue increase the appetite, making it difficult not to overeat. The body becomes depleted of its vital nutrients, so the adrenal glands are overworked. When this happens, we often crave a quick pick-up from caffeine or sugar.

- Body and mind can both be relaxed by exercise, but when under stress, people often stop their physical fitness programs because of the stress-related fatigue.

- And worst of all, it's difficult to maintain motivation when it seems that the program is no longer doing any good.

If you find yourself suffering from these reactions to stress, recognize that the problem does not lie with the program. The problem is that you're not allowing the program to work.

It's easy to say "relax," but much more difficult to do so. If you suffer from stress, you may wish to investigate self-hypnosis, which has helped many people learn how to achieve calm. Or you might find that the relaxation cassette tapes available at most health food stores can give you the assistance you need to unwind. But there are some simple steps you can begin right now to help you gain control over stress and minimize its destructive effects on your health. First of all, watch what you put into your body when you're under stress. Stop drinking coffee, tea, and caffeine-laden soft drinks, since they keep your inner mechanism working at high speed. Don't drink alcohol, either, since it produces a temporary, false feeling of relaxation, which is followed by even greater agitation. And avoid foods containing white sugar and white flour, since these substances agitate your body still further.

It is beneficial to increase your intake of B-complex vitamins, along with higher doses of pantothenic acid, niacinamide or niacin, Vitamin C and minerals—particularly calcium and magnesium. See Chapter 13 for suggested daily levels of vitamins and minerals when under stress.

Chiropractic care can also be very effective. Regular adjustments help to de-stress the body. Stress and tension build up in the neck and shoulder muscles as well as in the spine. A chiropractic adjustment will help to release the tightness and alleviate the pain.

There are several simple but effective techniques to bring your mind and body to a calmer state. Take several long, deep breaths, concentrating on slowly bringing the air into your lungs, and then slowly releasing it. One of our favorite ways to relieve stress is to stand on a mini-trampoline and bounce, ever so lightly, for about 5 minutes. Close your eyes and let the gentle up and down motion relax your tensed nerves. Or lie down, close your eyes, and picture a serene, happy place—perhaps a spot you visited on a recent vacation, or somewhere you've always dreamed of going. Take a few moments and picture the golden sands and turquoise water of an island paradise, or imagine the crunch of snow under your feet at a ski chalet. Let your mind wander away from the daily problems, and you'll return a few moments later in a more relaxed frame of mind.

We also recommend that you repeat the following affirmations to yourself whenever you're feeling particularly tense. Remember, you *can* get control over stress and you *can* quiet your thoughts and feelings, thus relaxing your body.

- I am free from tension, stress, and strain.

- I am feeling light, energized, and fully alive.

- Doubt and uncertainty have no power over me. I am assured of success.

- Love brings peace to my mind, body, and emotions. I love and accept myself just the way that I am.

10

EXERCISES NOT TO DO

When Franco was training for body-building competitions, he worked out 4 hours a day, doing a comprehensive program of weight training. Over the years, however, as he learned more and more about muscles and fat, and how various exercises work upon both, he realized that at least half of the exercises he had been doing were a total waste of time. He also realized that a number of standard exercises that are incorporated into most fitness routines have no real value. In fact, some of them can actually cause injuries.

Our purpose in this book is to help each woman find the weight-training and fitness program that will help her figure problems, while eliminating all of the time- and energy-consuming exercises that do nothing to promote health and fitness.

How many of these exercises have you done assuming they do great things for you?

Head Stands
Twisting with a Bar Behind the Neck or Back
Good Mornings
Jumping Jacks
Bench Squat
Roman Chair Sit-Ups
Sit-Ups with Hands Clasped Behind Head or Neck
Quadriceps Stretch
Seated Stretch with Knees Bent
Wide-Grip Bench Press
Standing Side Bends with Weights
Standing Reverse Barbell Curls

Many of these are exercises you learned in school. Who doesn't remember being in a squad of gym-suited 14-year-olds doing 50 jumping jacks, with the teacher counting faster and faster? Learning why jumping jacks and other such movements expend valuable energy while doing nothing to help your body will give you a better understanding of how your body works and how to take the best possible care of it.

By eliminating useless or dangerous exercises from your workouts and substituting effective alternatives, you'll achieve better results in less time.

A DOZEN USELESS EXERCISES

- HEAD STANDS. This exercise causes compression of the cervical spine, which can produce such problems as headaches and neck, shoulder, or arm pain.

- TWISTING. There is a common misconception that twisting with a bar or stick behind the neck or back reduces the fat from the sides of the waist, but nothing could be further from the truth. Muscles can only stretch or contract. As you can see from the diagram, muscles on the sides, back, and front of the waist run in a vertical direction. They should stretch and contract in that same direction. Twisting, particularly with a bar or stick, forces the muscle to extend itself in an unnatural manner. Not only is the exercise ineffective for reducing fat, but it also can cause permanent spinal problems. Just look at the unnatural motion called for in this exercise and you'll see what we mean.

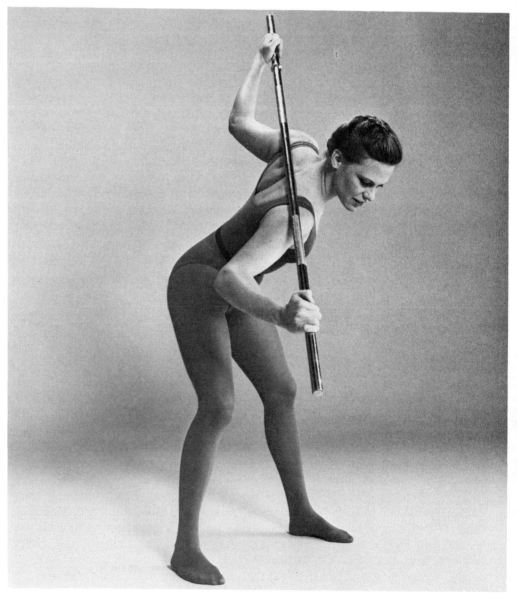

Don't

The neck turns 90 degrees, or a quarter rotation, while the lower back is forced forward and in a 35-degree sideways motion that is exaggerated by the swing of the stick. This movement can damage the lumbar area of the spine, and even cause traumatic arthritis. It can also cause the muscles to go into spasm, pulling the vertebrae out of alignment. In addition, doing this ineffective, potentially harmful exercise takes time and energy away from those that are beneficial.

- GOOD MORNINGS. These are forward bends with a bar across the shoulders, done with straight knees. The exercises can cause the lower spine to go out of alignment, as well as compressing the nerves of the shoulders and arms. They are of some benefit in stretching the hamstring muscles, but we have an alternative that does the same thing without the drawbacks of this exercise. (See pages 42–45 for the hamstring stretch.)

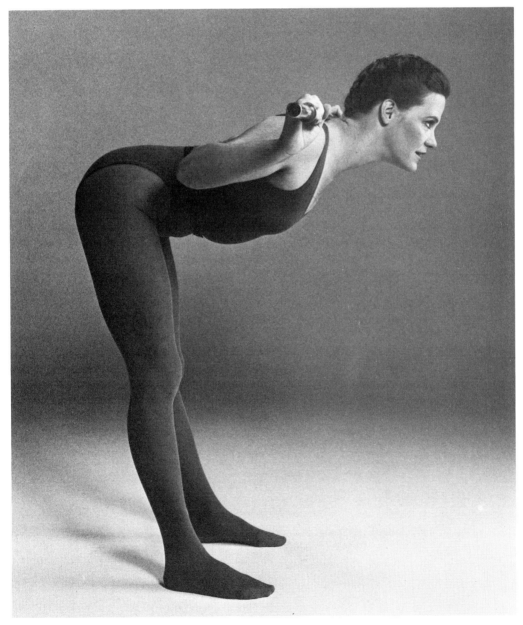

Don't

- JUMPING JACKS. A popular exercise that has been in use for years, jumping jacks do nothing for the body. In fact, the constant jolting causes compression of all the weight-bearing joints (ankles, knees, hips), resulting in nerve blockage to the extremities. For women there are additional dangers, since continual jumping, like jogging, can cause the uterus to slip out of place and can weaken the muscles supporting the breasts, making them sag. Muscle tests performed on subjects who have just completed a vigorous set of jumping jacks indicate a general loss of strength. Nor does the exercise do anything to improve the cardiovascular system.

- BENCH SQUAT. This is similar to a regular squat, except that the hips touch the bench. It is frequently used by both men and women power lifters under the mistaken impression that it increases strength for the regular squat. In fact, it increases disk compression, which in turn diminishes the nerve supply to the leg muscles, thus weakening the legs.

- ROMAN CHAIR SIT-UPS. Although commonly used in many exercise programs, this is the least effective stomach exercise. The stomach is improved only when the abdominal muscles are directly involved in the movement. As you can see from the photo, the iliopsoas, or lower back, muscles are doing most of the work, not the abdominals. This movement can also cause muscle spasms in the lower back, which can pull the lower thoracic and lumbar vertebrae out of alignment.

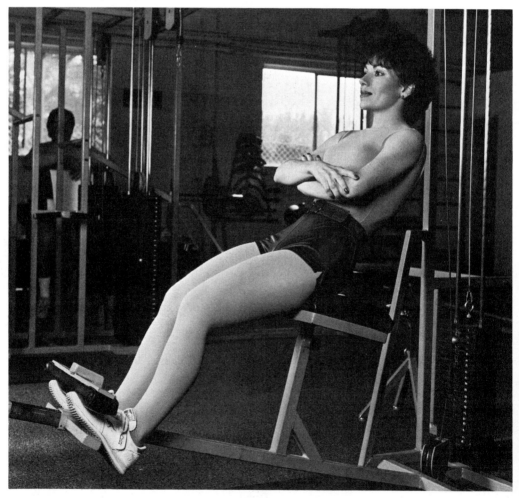

Don't

- SIT-UPS WITH HANDS CLASPED BEHIND THE HEAD OR NECK. Although used in many gym and home-exercise programs, this exercise forces the neck to be held at an angle that can actually weaken neck muscles, contributing to poor posture and even stressing the muscles that control the jaw. Sit-ups should be done with the hands placed on the chest, with the abdominals doing the work.

- QUADRICEPS STRETCH. Runners in particular frequently stretch the quadriceps, the large muscle that runs along the front of the thigh. This exercise is unnecessary because this muscle is stretched every time the knee is bent—every time we sit down, for instance. When one muscle is overstretched it becomes weaker than usual. Extra stretching of the quadriceps can weaken other muscles along the front of the leg, creating an imbalance in the musculature that can cause knee problems—particularly for women.

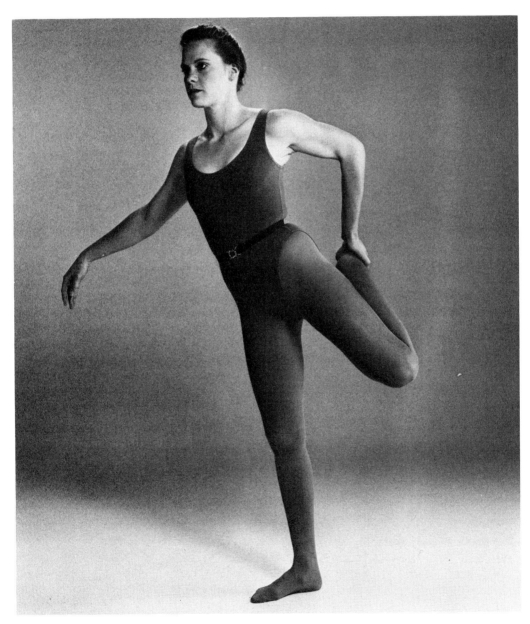

Don't

153

· SEATED STRETCH WITH KNEES BENT. Besides causing all the problems of the quadriceps stretch, this exercise can also stretch ligaments in the knee, leading to possible cartilage problems. Since ligaments stabilize the joints, they must always be tight. The exercise does nothing to trim, firm, or slim your body, either.

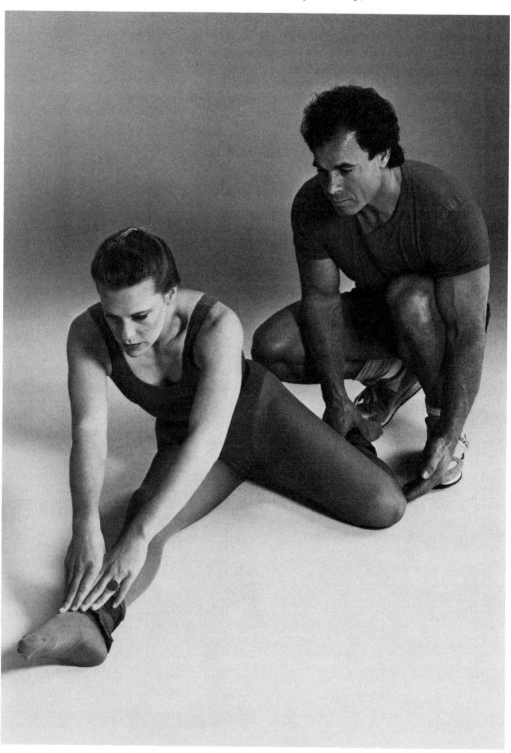

Don't

- WIDE-GRIP BENCH PRESS. A wide grip produces abnormal leverage during the bench press, which contributes to injuries to the front of the shoulders. We recommend a medium grip (about 30 to 35 inches between the hands), which is more beneficial in developing muscle strength and fitness.

- STANDING SIDE BENDS WITH WEIGHTS. This exercise does exactly the opposite of what you're trying to accomplish; it thickens and shortens the large muscles at the side of the waist, which actually makes the waist larger, besides contributing to an abnormal curvature of the spine. To reduce body fat around the waist, side bends are effective only when done *without* weights.

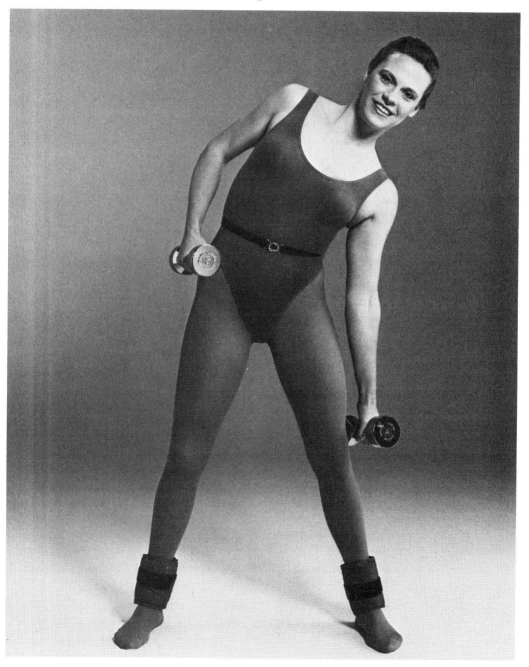

Don't

- STANDING REVERSE BARBELL CURLS. This exercise is not only ineffective in reducing body fat and increasing muscle strength, it also contributes to tennis elbow and shoulder problems. The forearm bones and muscles are rotated and do not move freely in this exercise, resulting in a movement too limited to be effective. Shoulder problems can occur because the exercise twists the biceps and forces the shoulder back in an unnatural manner.

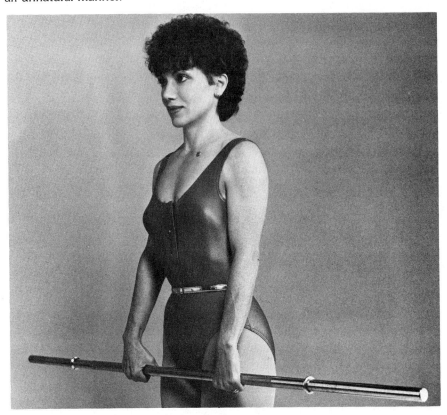

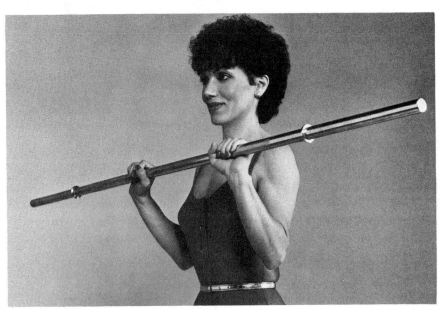

Don't

11

POSTURE AND INJURIES

Actors and actresses often say that they're able to capture the essence of the personalities they portray by envisioning the way the characters would walk and stand. Posture swiftly and dramatically communicates a great deal about a person. With just a glance at how a woman is standing, you can usually tell how she is feeling—if she is self-confident, if she likes her body, if she is healthy, or if her little toe hurts.

Look in the mirror. What does your posture tell the world about you? Does it convey self-confidence, energy, and enthusiasm? Or does an unattractive slouch indicate low self-esteem and lack of vitality? And does your poor posture make you look at least 10 pounds heavier than you actually are?

We've all seen those magazine and newspaper ads raving about instant weight-loss pills or machines, and flaunting "before" and "after" pictures taken hours or days later. The real reason those models look "instantly" better, though, is that their posture is better. Look back to Chapter 2 and see how our "before" and "after" women have improved their posture and trimmed their bodies through exercise. The combination of spot-reducing and posture exercises results in the most dramatic changes possible in the shortest amount of time. Take a look at the pictures of Alison in Chapter 2. Notice that even though her weight loss was not great, the changes in her posture and the shape of her body make her look at least 20 pounds thinner.

No matter how trim and fit you become, you're simply not going to look and feel your best without good posture. As well as giving you a graceful, attractive appearance, standing, walking, and sitting correctly prevents undue strain on muscles, joints and ligaments. Many of the patients we treat in our chiropractic practice suffer from the aches and pains that directly result from poor posture. When they learn to stand, walk, and sit correctly, they look better *and* feel better.

Understanding the basics of good posture means understanding something about your spine. Besides serving as the support for your torso, the spine is your body's communication center; impulses travel through it from the brain to the nerves and muscles. This complex and delicate skeletal system is made up of vertebrae, which are like separate but interlocking bricks, stacked on top of each other. In between each "brick" is a disk, which absorbs the jolts caused by everyday movement—jolts that otherwise could easily shock the vertebrae out of alignment.

In many women, the body is thrown out of proper alignment by poor posture, muscles weakened by lack of exercise, and too much extra weight. This can put undue pressure on the nerves, resulting in painful and frequently debilitating back pain.

Fortunately, in most cases poor posture is just a bad habit. Like any other bad habit, it can be broken, with concentration and self-reminders.

Practice standing, sitting, bending, and lifting correctly, and you'll eliminate a major cause of back trouble. Remember that whether you are working or playing, asleep or awake, your muscles are supporting you. Weight training is important, positive action that will help make you constantly aware of good posture. Working with weights will help you to strengthen the muscles, tendons, and ligaments that hold your spine in place.

The exercises listed in this section will strengthen the muscles in your back and reinforce your best posture.

EXERCISES FOR BETTER POSTURE

Upper Back

These exercises, which can be done at home with free weights, strengthen the upper back muscles to hold the body more erect. This is particularly important for women who spend their days at desk jobs, since prolonged sitting weakens the upper back.

DO 3 SETS OF 20 REPS, 3 TIMES PER WEEK

- Bent-Over Lateral Raises (See pages 56–57)
- One-Arm Rowing (See page 55)
- Barbell Rowing (See page 73)

Lower Back

Lower back problems are probably the most common chiropractic problem we encounter in our practice. Once again, sitting for prolonged periods is extremely harmful, since it causes compression of the vertebrae, thus intensifying lower back problems. Prevention of such problems should include exercises to strengthen the lower back and stretch the hamstring muscles. The following exercises are most effective for those purposes.

DO 3 SETS OF 20 REPS, 3 TIMES PER WEEK

- Pulldowns in Front of the Neck (See page 138)
- Barbell Rowing (See page 73)
- One-Arm Rowing (See page 55)
- Hamstring Stretch (See pages 42–45)
- Hyperextension: Lie on your stomach and raise your head and torso, as shown. Stretch the head and neck back, so that you are looking at the ceiling. Hold for one minute.

Neck

Neck and shoulder problems are quite common in women, in whom stress is often reflected in tightened muscles in this area. Many women too have neck problems from incorrect abdominal exercises (such as doing sit-ups with hands behind the head or neck), sleeping on pillows that are too high, sitting in a hunched-over position at a desk, or from injuries, such as whiplash. Neck tension also contributes to headaches. We recommend a program that includes one exercise for strength and one stretch to relieve the strain.

- Anterior Neck Lift
- Lateral Neck Stretch

Exercise 79: Anterior Neck Lift

Lie on the floor with a pillow under your neck. Raise your head as shown. Don't bring the head all the way to the chest. Then return to starting position, and repeat.

Do 3 sets of 10 reps.

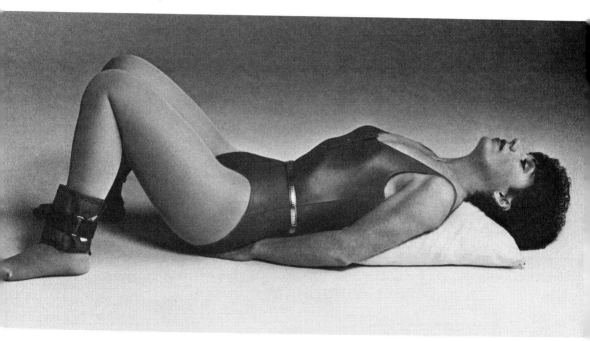

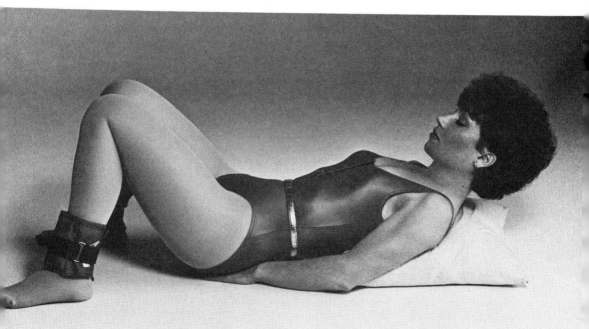

Exercise 80: Lateral Neck Stretch

Bend your neck as if trying to touch ear to shoulder. Then, using the hand on the same side of the body, gently pull the head closer to the shoulder. Hold the stretch for 1 minute.

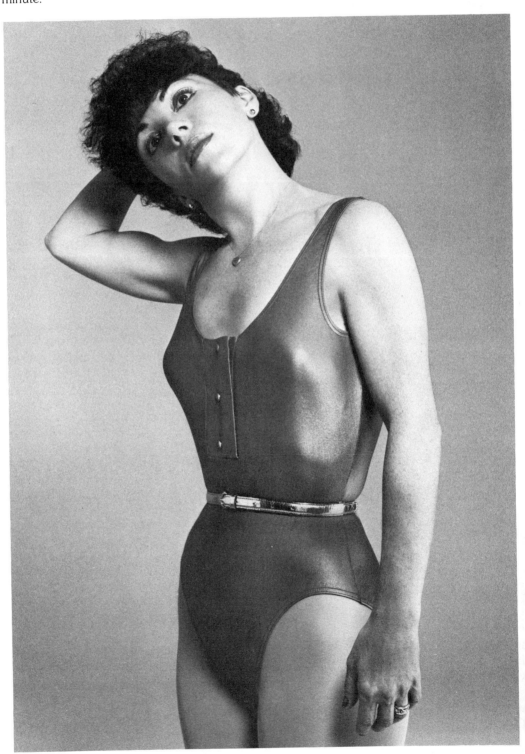

The Entire Spine

One of the most serious problems resulting from poor posture is compression of the spine. Hanging by your hands with knees bent helps to decompress the spine. Hang for a few minutes from a chinning bar or by holding on to the top of an open door. Hang twice a day, morning and evening, for 2 to 3 minutes.

INJURIES

Most exercise injuries can be avoided by using common sense and some preventive exercises. There are also some simple movements you can do to help you recover more quickly from many of the minor injuries you might sustain.

Prevention

Stretching properly before exercising is the best insurance against injury. As we discussed in Chapter 4, stretching helps prepare the body for your strenuous routine. Chest, biceps, calf, and especially hamstring muscles all need to be systematically stretched before any workout to prevent muscle strains and other injuries.

While stretching is beneficial in all sports and exercise programs, it is especially necessary in weight training, which tends to make muscles tighter as well as stronger. Be sure to devote special attention and time to the hamstring muscles, which must be properly stretched to avoid injuries throughout the lower body, including the back, hip, knee, and ankle.

To prevent injuries while weight training, here are some common sense rules to follow:

- Warm up before each session. Be sure to stretch the flexor muscles, which are probably the tightest: the calves, hamstrings, obliques, chest, biceps, upper trapezius, and the anterior forearm.

- Have a good grip on the weights. If your grip is not secure, put the weights down and begin again.

- Don't try to do more than you are ready to do. You can't switch from a pair of 5-pound dumbbells to a 25-pound set without increasing your risk of injury. Be patient and allow your body to increase its strength gradually

- Do a full range of controlled motion with each move.

How to Tell When You're Injured

Many beginning weight trainers report that they don't know how to tell the difference between ordinary muscle soreness and actual injury. While soreness is to be expected when beginning a strenuous weight-training program, you can distinguish it from injury by the intensity and the duration of the pain. Soreness generally begins the day after exercising, lasts from 3 to 5 days, and is felt throughout a particular body area. Injuries are felt immediately, with highly localized pain that can last indefinitely.

For soreness, we recommend large doses of Vitamin C—1000 mg up to 5 or 6 times a day. It's also important to drink 6 to 8 glasses of water a day, which flushes toxins out of the system. Hot baths or showers also help reduce muscle soreness.

Injuries should be treated by a professional.

Muscle Cramps

It is not unusual to experience occasional, brief muscle cramps when doing strenuous exercise. If you suffer from frequent, prolonged cramping, however, you should recognize it as a warning signal that you are not taking proper care of your body. We have found that the most common cause of abnormal cramping is poor nutrition, usually a severe calcium/magnesium deficiency. Women who go on crash diets, hoping to speed up their body transformation, often suffer from severe and prolonged muscle cramps. We recommend attention to well-balanced nutrition, especially when you're trying to lose weight (see Chapter 13 on nutrition).

To function properly, muscles need a sufficient supply of calcium and magnesium, which are often missing in many diets, particularly those heavy on protein. Liquid or capsule supplements of these minerals will help if your prolonged cramping is caused by a deficiency in your diet.

Muscle Spasms

While not as severe as cramps, muscle spasms can be longer in duration and, in some cases, can even become chronic. Spasms are involuntary tightening and shortening of the muscles and have a variety of causes, including improper training, poor nutrition, and emotional stress.

To prevent spasms, be sure to use common sense in your weight-training exercises.

- Don't use weights that are too heavy for you to handle comfortably.

- Keep weights properly balanced to avoid uneven pressure on various body parts.

- Always warm up thoroughly.

- Maintain good nutrition. (See Chapter 13.) Remember that sugar is your muscles' worst enemy. Large doses of sugar sharply raise the blood-sugar level, which immediately drops again to a point lower than normal, leaving you weaker and your muscles more vulnerable.

- As with muscle cramps, we have found that calcium/magnesium supplements in liquid or capsule form are helpful in maintaining muscle strength and well-being and preventing spasms.

- Approach your weight training with a clear, relaxed frame of mine. Everyday tension should be left behind when you pick up your weights, or you'll increase the risk of muscle contraction, spasms, cramps, and injuries. Use stretching warm-ups to ease your mind and body into your daily program.

- Apply an ice cube directly to a muscle that is beginning to spasm, rubbing the cube on the area for 5 to 7 minutes. Repeat several times a day. If the spasm has not gone away after a day or two, use moist—never dry—heat in the form of a moist heating pad, hot water bottle, hot shower, or bath.

Strains and Sprains

These two types of injuries are similar, except that strains involve muscles, tendons and their attachments, while sprains involve ligaments.

If you suspect that you have a serious strain or sprain, see your doctor.

Muscle strains are generally caused by overuse or overstress, and are fairly common among weight trainers who overtrain. To avoid these injuries:

- Don't train when you're tired. Most injuries occur when a person is already exhausted but wants to complete "just one more set."

- Don't overtrain. Learn the symptoms of overtraining, and listen to your body.

- Always warm up thoroughly.

- Reduce—or, better yet, completely eliminate—processed sugar from your diet.

- Never let your mind wander while you are training. At all times you must concentrate on what you're doing, not only to achieve the desired results, but also to avoid injuries.

Sprains are injuries to a joint that cause severe pain and loss of movement. Symptoms include rapid swelling, bruising or skin discoloration, loss or restriction of motion, and a sensation of heat around the injured joint. If a sprain occurs, immediately apply ice with a circular motion for 5 to 7 minutes several times a day. A body support such as an Ace bandage may be needed while the body heals.

To prevent sprains:

- Warm up and warm down properly.

- Avoid overtraining.

- Do not do any movements that feel unnatural or uncomfortable.

When we see patients with strains and sprains, we always recommend the same formula: R.I.C.E. That's Rest, Ice, Compression, and Elevation. Your body needs time to heal, so REST. Heat will cause too much blood to flow to the injured area, resulting in increased swelling, so use ICE. After 48 hours, applying heat to the muscle will often aid healing. Wrapping the area reduces swelling so use COMPRESSION (but never apply a bandage too tightly). Propping the injured area on a chair or table or with pillows aids in fluid drainage and also decreases the swelling, so use ELEVATION.

Bursitis

Bursae are sacs or cavities of lubricating fluid that protect the joints or tendons. Bursitis is an extremely painful condition caused by swelling of the bursae, particularly in the shoulder, elbow, knee, and ankle areas. If you suspect bursitis, contact your doctor, and in the meantime use moist heat on the swollen area for 10 to 15 minutes, 2 to 3 times daily. Avoid training the affected area until it heals.

To prevent bursitis, avoid overexercising any given area, since this condition tends to occur when too many exercises are done involving the same joint.

Fractures

Always see your doctor immediately if you suspect you have suffered a fracture. Symptoms of a broken bone include swelling, bruising or discoloration, and intense pain. Untreated fractures can result in permanent disability as well as nerve, muscle, and blood vessel damage.

Varicose Veins

These are blood vessels, usually in the legs, that are abnormally dilated, knotted, or twisted. Proper nutrition, including vitamin and mineral supplements (vitamins B-6, E, and C as well as calcium/magnesium), is often helpful. The tendency to varicose veins is inherited, but that doesn't mean you have to let them develop. There are preventive measures:

- Stay at your ideal weight.

- Get plenty of exercise, especially exercise that encourages good circulation in the lower part of the body.

- Avoid tight clothes, undergarments, or boots that might inhibit circulation. Support hose, of course, will help by reducing the pressure on the veins in your legs.

- Avoid crossing the legs at the knee, which inhibits proper circulation.

- Elevate your feet whenever you have the opportunity.

If you do develop varicose veins and they become swollen, apply ice packs on the affected areas.

Shinsplints

Just about every beginning runner has spent at least a few days hobbling from the pain of shinsplints. This debilitating injury is a result of an imbalance between the anterior (shin) and posterior calf muscles: The front muscle is weak and the back muscle is too tight. To prevent—and treat—this disability, stretch the posterior calf muscles well before each exercise period. Strengthen the anterior muscles by placing the heels on a block and raising the toes as high as possible. Then lower as far as possible. Do 3 sets of 20 reps. Stretch the calf muscles by doing calf raises: Place the toes on a step or block and lower the heels as far as possible. Lift, and repeat. Do 3 sets of 20 reps.

A Note About Gravity Machines

Among the more popular exercise and fitness machines these days are the antigravity machines, which allow the user to hang upside down by the thighs or ankles, improving circulation to the upper extremities while reducing pressure and compression on the spine caused by everyday activities. They are often used to treat back injuries.

The gravity-traction machines use gravity to reverse the spinal compression that occurs every time we stand, sit, or walk, in addition to increasing the disk spaces between the vertebrae. Many of our patients find relief from muscle spasm, back and leg pain, and tension after hanging on an antigravity machine. There are several different types of antigravity systems currently available, but we prefer one that permits hanging by the thighs, as shown in the illustration. In our opinion, hanging by the ankles causes stress to the ligaments of the ankle, knee, and hip, in addition to weakening the muscles that support the lower back.

While hanging from the ankles is generally beneficial for those with sway-back (lordotic curvature), gravity machines should be prescribed by a professional who thoroughly understands spinal mechanics. The type of machine recommended should be suited to the patient's structure as shown on spinal X-rays. These machines are not beneficial for every physical condition, and should not be recommended for everyone.

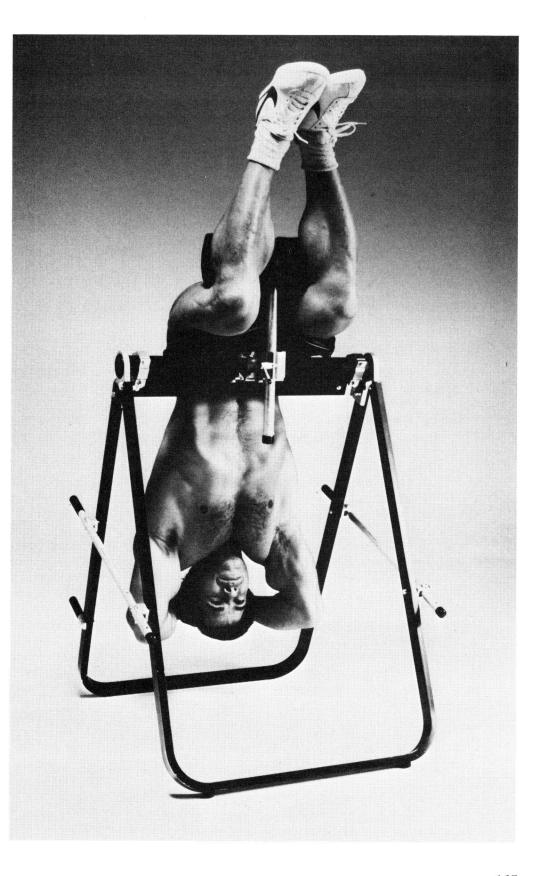

12

WEIGHT TRAINING FOR OTHER SPORTS

Although participating in sports is far healthier than sitting in front of the television munching chips, sports alone will not solve your weight and figure problems. Like other forms of exercise, sports raise your basic metabolic rate, thus increasing the amount of oxygen in your blood and enabling your body to burn more calories. Sports are good for releasing tension and can improve agility and stamina. Combined with weight training, they provide a balanced approach to physical fitness.

But sports are games. True, they're usually very active games, but they can't give you a complete body workout or systematically improve strength and flexibility. And nearly every sport carries some risk of injury.

No sport can equal aerobic weight training in providing all-around fitness. It is a full-body equalizer, strengthening and firming where the body needs it, zeroing in on individual muscle groups. But sports and games do provide enjoyable, competitive social activity that is part of a well-balanced approach to physical fitness. To get the most enjoyment and the greatest physical benefit from your sports hobbies, it's important to do some weight-training exercises to strengthen the areas that are most vulnerable to injury. Warming up before playing is also good common sense.

You'll notice some other benefits as you begin to combine weight training with your usual sports activities. Your improved muscle strength and flexibility will increase your endurance and allow you to move faster and with greater agility. Of course, carrying around less stored body fat will improve your performance, no matter which sport you engage in.

Many people go limping into the office on Monday mornings because they don't know how to use their bodies correctly during their weekend sports workouts. Tennis can produce sore knees and elbows. Running can wreak havoc with knees and internal organs. Bicycling can produce tremendous strain on shoulders and back. Don't cut out these activities—their plusses far outweigh their minuses. If you enjoy them, make them an integral part of your overall fitness scheme. But do use weight training in combination with your favorite sports; by strengthening muscles, you'll prevent injuries.

As with everything in life, each sport has its assets and liabilities. Our purpose is to help you prepare to get the most benefit and enjoyment out of the ones you choose. In other words, let's maximize the assets and minimize the liabilities.

AEROBIC EXERCISE

This activity is beginning to eclipse even running as the "in" exercise for men as well as women. Aerobic classes provide definite benefits in cardiovascular conditioning, improving circulation, and increasing the metabolic rate. It reduces stress, aids in digestion, and can work wonders in breaking down fat tissue. But many people hobble away from aerobic classes with knee, ankle, and lower back pain. Stress fractures can also occur, and after prolonged aerobic sessions some women suffer from prolapses of vital organs, i.e., their uterus or bladder slips out of place. And while aerobics are great for shaping up and spot reducing your lower body, they don't do much for bulges above the waist.

Don't give up your aerobic workouts. Enjoy them, but eliminate the jumping and bouncing that can be so harmful to joints and internal organs. Aim for smooth, flowing movements. Remember the rapid movements we suggest you use in weight training? Bring that same sort of controlled motion to the aerobics class, and you'll be kind to your body while you're reshaping your figure. Concentrate on using your abdominal muscles to support movement in the lower torso, and remember not to arch your back, or you'll do it permanent harm. When doing leg movements, remember to flex and lift, to initiate the motions from the hip joint rather than the knee, and avoid twists and sharp turns. During exercise, concentrate on keeping muscles taut and movements smooth.

Don't forget to warm up and warm down adequately before and after each session. (See Chapter 4 for good pre- and post-aerobics stretches. The exercises in Program I done with 3-pound ankle weights will strengthen your muscles, increase your endurance, and help to prevent injuries in aerobics class.)

BASKETBALL

You don't have to be Kareem Abdul-Jabbar to get a good workout from basketball. The combination of running up and down the court, jumping, shooting, and dodging provides good general conditioning while burning 300 to 600 calories per hour. Knees, ankles, and lower back are particularly vulnerable in this sport, so if you play basketball regularly, do the advanced home or gym program twice a week to increase strength and flexibility in these areas. As in tennis, racquetball, badminton, and volleyball, try to keep your body moving constantly in the eventual direction of the ball, so that you won't rely on a dangerous lunge at the last minute. Avoid abrupt twisting motions of the knees and ankles.

To reduce on-court muscle fatigue in your lower body, do the stretching exercises listed in Chapter 4. For the upper body, the Seated Neck Press will increase strength and endurance, particularly in throwing, passing, and shooting:

Sit on your bench or a stool and hold a 20- to 30-pound barbell behind your head, above your neck. Extend the arms until they are completely straight. Return to original position. Do 3 sets of 10 reps, twice a week.

BICYCLING

Biking burns from 450 to 900 calories per hour and is terrific for working the legs and improving the cardiovascular system. It does virtually nothing for the upper body, however, and the hunched-shoulder posture can result in improper breathing and poor circulation as well as muscle strain in the neck and upper back.

Try to keep your upper body as loose and relaxed as possible when cycling. Make certain the bike fits you properly. The seat should be just high enough to allow a good stretch for your legs, but your knees should never be completely straight.

To improve your cycling strength and endurance, do the upper body exercises from the split program for home or gym.

BOWLING

Bowling provides a good workout for your legs, but involves imbalanced movements in the upper body. Compensating exercises are needed to improve wrist and arm strength, and to loosen leg muscles, which are moved tightly and sporadically in this sport, which burns from 150 to 200 calories per hour.

All-over body stretches are a must before bowling, as well as the preacher's curl (see page 136), which develops the forearm. Front raises (see page 111) will help develop the shoulder muscles that increase the power of your throw. Leg extensions will strengthen the quadriceps, which can get a workout in the game.

GOLF

A less strenuous sport than tennis or running, golf uses from 240 to 300 calories per hour. While beneficial to the lower body, it doesn't provide the same all-over conditioning and cardiovascular benefits as tennis or aerobics. Just because it's less strenuous, however, doesn't mean there aren't still opportunities for injury. Elbow, upper back, knee, and ankle injuries can occur if you're not properly conditioned. Before starting to play, warm up by holding the golf club in the hand you ordinarily don't use, and reverse your normal swing. Repeat this activity for about 5 minutes before and after each game.

Also beneficial is the Dumbbell Swing, which improves power, loosens back muscles, and increases arm strength and flexibility:

Standing with your feet slightly apart, grip a 20-pound dumbbell with both hands. Then swing the dumbbell down to the floor, bending the knees. Bring arms up to the original position. Do 2 sets of 12 reps 3 times a week.

We also recommend the upper body exercises in the split program for home or gym.

HIKING, CLIMBING, AND BACKPACKING

While hiking, climbing, and backpacking are particularly good for the lower body, they also provide fairly effective cardiovascular conditioning while burning 300 to 600 calories per hour. The advanced home or gym program is ideal for building up the strength, endurance, and flexibility necessary for these often strenuous outdoor activities. In addition, backpackers may wish to incorporate the Clean and Press into their program, since it conditions the entire body while doing wonders to increase upper body strength:

Standing with feet slightly apart and knees bent, grasp the barbell using the over handgrip. Straighten the knees and bring the barbell up to shoulder height. Then lift it directly overhead. Return it to shoulder level, then to the floor. Using 20 to 40 pounds, do 3 sets of 12 reps, twice a week.

HORSEBACK RIDING

While the horse is getting a great aerobic workout, you're primarily exercising your quadriceps, hamstrings, and gluteus muscles. To firm and strengthen the rest of your body, you need to combine horseback riding with aerobic exercises such as running, swimming, or jumping rope.

It's of crucial importance to stretch the hamstring muscle (see pages 42–45) before and after horseback riding. Most of the back problems associated with horseback riding come from inadequately stretched hamstrings.

In addition, the upper body exercises from Program I will balance the workout the lower part of your body gets from horseback riding. Do the program at least twice a week if you ride regularly.

RUNNING

There's no argument about the benefits of running: It improves the cardiovascular system, provides all-over conditioning, and reduces, tightens, and firms the hips and buttocks while firming the calves. But running has its drawbacks. Knees and hamstring muscles are often casualties of a running program that doesn't compensate for the strain placed upon those areas. Improper shoulder and arm movements can hamper correct breathing and cause muscle tension in the upper back. While it burns from 450 to 750 calories per hour and does wonders for your legs, running doesn't do much for the middle body. In addition, runners usually need to build up the upper body with weights in order to increase the glycogen storage capacity, because it is used up in tremendous quantities during long distance runs. Always precede your running with warm-ups, placing special emphasis on stretching the hamstrings and calves (see Chapter 4). When running, be sure to relax your shoulders and allow your arms to swing naturally. Use a gliding motion, or alternate between fast running and fast walking, a motion which doesn't compress the joints.

Dumbbell Calf Raises shape and firm your legs while increasing your running stamina:

Stand holding onto the back of a chair, the right foot resting on a 3-inch block or book and the left leg bent. Holding a 5- to 10-pound dumbbell in your right hand, rise up and down on your toes. After completing the required repetitions, change legs. Do 1 set of 15 reps with each leg for the first 2 weeks, then increase to 2 sets of 15 for 2 weeks, working up to 3 sets of 20.

Jogging is one of the few sports we never recommend. It is a slow, up and down bouncing movement rather than a fast, gliding motion. Jogging jolts the weight-bearing joints in much the same way that aerobic classes do and can compress the spine, upset internal organs, and cause loss of muscle elasticity. Run. Walk. Don't jog.

For runners, we recommend the series of upper body exercises from the split program for home or gym. Do this upper body program at least twice a week.

SKATING

A healthful, fun way to get where you're going—and to get some exercise—skating is an excellent conditioning exercise that uses from 300 to 600 calories per hour. Skating improves flexibility and cardiovascular capacity, and is helpful in trimming the lower body. Since the smooth, graceful movements of skating are less stressful than jogging, this is an excellent exercise to use as an alternate on days when you are not training with weights.

To strengthen the quadriceps, leg extensions are very effective. Do 5 sets of 20 reps.

The Leg Press is a gym exercise that is particularly good for developing strong hip and thigh muscles, which are needed skating:

> Sit at the leg press machine with your feet pressing the pedals. Exhale as you push, inhale as you return to the starting position. You may use either your toes or your entire foot, whichever feels comfortable. Do 3 sets of 8 reps.

SKIING

The exhilaration and beautiful natural setting of skiing make this sport one of the most enjoyable ways to burn from 360 to 900 calories per hour. Whether downhill or cross-country, skiing provides an excellent workout for your entire body, increases flexibility, and improves the cardiovascular system. Unfortunately, it can also result in injuries, particularly to the knee and ankle joints.

To increase flexibility, improve stamina and reduce the chance of injuries, do the following exercises 3 to 4 times a week.

EXERCISE	SETS	REPS
Triceps Pushdowns	4	15
Squats	3	25
Lunges	3	25
Leg Extensions	5	30
Pulldowns	3	25

Do the following stretches before and after skiing to prevent injuries:

Oblique Stretch	1 minute
Hamstring Stretch	1 minute
Calf Stretch	1 minute

An excellent pre-skiing leg exercise you can do at the gym is the leg extension (shown on page 96). Start with 5 sets of 15 reps using 30 pounds. Build up to 5 sets of 30 reps using 40 to 50 pounds.

Cross-country skiers will benefit from squats, which improve balance and strengthen the muscles around the hip and knee joints. See the description of barbell squats on page 74. Using 30- to 50-pound barbells, do 4 sets of 12 reps, 2 or 3 times each week.

SOFTBALL

Though not the most effective sport for burning calories (only about 250 per hour) or reducing body fat, softball is fun and provides a good tone-up for the lower body and moderate conditioning for the upper body. Since quick movements from a standing position are often called for, knee and ankle injuries are common.

The upper body exercises from Program I will strengthen those areas, and should be done twice a week. In addition, warm up thoroughly prior to each session, using the stretches listed in Chapter 4.

To increase dramatically your throwing and hitting power, try adding the Close-Grip Bench Press to your regular weight-training routine:

> *Lie on your back with the barbell held in an overhand grip, arms bent with the barbell at chest height. Raise the barbell until your arms are straight. Return the weight to your chest. Repeat. Using 15 to 25 pounds, do 4 sets of 10 reps, twice a week.*

SWIMMING

An excellent sport for improving all-over conditioning, flexibility, and coordination, swimming is the perfect exercise to balance your weight training. Using from 360 to 720 calories per hour, swimming is an ideal exercise for women of all ages and body types.

Even though injuries are less likely in this fluid, graceful sport, they can still occur if your muscles are not trained to compensate for the movements required in the pool. For example, lower back muscles, which can be strained when doing the backstroke, should be strengthened with the Modified Push-Up:

> *Lie flat on the floor on your stomach, with arms bent and your palms flat on the floor at chest level. Raise your head and upper body until your arms are straight. Lower your body to the floor. Do this exercise daily: 2 sets of 10 reps.*

You'll strengthen your shoulders and improve your aquatic endurance by incorporating the following exercise into your weight-training program:

Upright Rowing.
> *Stand straight and, using the overhand grip, place your hands 6 inches apart on a 20- to 30-pound barbell. Pull the bar up to your chin; hold; then lower it to thigh level. Repeat. Do 3 sets of 10 reps twice a week.*

TENNIS

Tennis is wonderful for improving your concentration while producing all-over body conditioning. The mental attitude required for this fast-moving sport is great for reducing tension and anxiety. And everybody needs to release a little aggression sometimes! An energetic set of tennis gets your heart and blood moving, trims legs, hips, and buns.

But it can also lead to a variety of injuries, particularly in women, who generally have less upper body strength than men. To reduce the risk of getting hurt, warm up thoroughly before each session. Ten minutes of stretching exercises (see Chapter 4) will pay off in greater agility on the court and less soreness after the game. When playing, try to use the strength of your shoulder and back to put power into your shots rather than making your arm do all the work. Keep the shoulder, elbow, and wrist stable, and using small steps, keep moving in the direction of the ball instead of relying on last-minute lunges to take you across the court. When serving the ball or standing in place, keep your feet slightly apart, in line with your hips.

To get the most from your tennis workout without paying a high price in aches and pains afterward, we recommend the following exercises to strengthen the upper body, particularly the upper back, shoulders, triceps, and forearm. Do these exercises 3 times a week, along with daily stretching, and you'll not only minimize the chance of tennis elbow and hamstring strains, but your increased upper-body strength will also improve your game. In fact, you'll probably even be able to add the one-handed backhand to your repertoire.

EXERCISE	SETS	REPS
One-Arm Rowing	3	15
Bent-Over Lateral Raises	3	15
Lateral Raises	3	15
Lying Triceps Extension	4	15
Dumbbell Curls	4	15
Hamstring Stretch	1	1 minute
Trapezius Stretch	1	1 minute

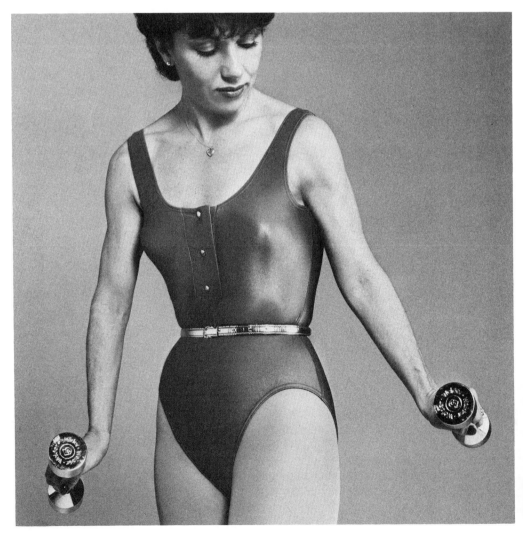

Oblique Stretch with Weights	1	1 minute
Forearm Extension & Flexion	3	15

Forearm Extension and Flexion is used to prevent and improve tennis elbow problems. Do the exercise exactly as shown 3 times per week. Hold 3–5-pound dumbbell in each hand. Extend wrist out for 15 reps and then in for 15 reps.

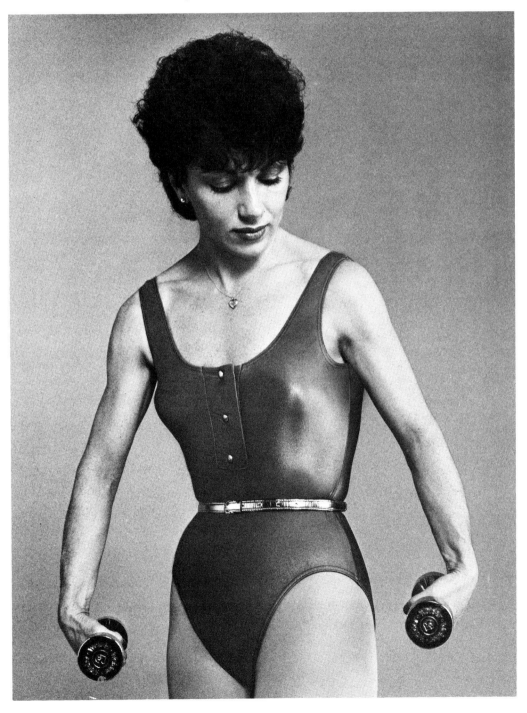

VOLLEYBALL

You'll notice trimmer hips and thighs, firmer arms, and improved cardiovascular capacity after regular games of volleyball. You'll also be burning 300 to 600 calories per hour. As with the other sports incorporating quick movements, you'll need to strengthen your legs and ankles to reduce the risk of injuries.

Do the advanced program for home or gym twice a week as preventive measures, always warming up first with the stretches in Chapter 4.

To improve the back and upper-arm strength so essential for spiking the ball, do the Bent-Over Barbell Rowing exercise twice each week:

> *Holding the barbell in an overhand grip, bend over from the waist and fully extend the arms, letting the barbell hang. Then still bending over, raise it to your chest. Lower and raise again. Do 3 sets of 10 reps, with a 20- to 30-pound weight.*

13

NUTRITION

The exercises in this book will help reshape your body, but without sound nutrition, you won't achieve optimum results, and you certainly won't maintain your beautiful new body. Good nutrition is the foundation of health, strength, and beauty. Don't believe anyone who tells you they're in great shape on a regular diet of junk food. It simply isn't true.

To stay in top physical condition, your body needs a balanced diet of protein, carbohydrates, fat, vitamins, minerals, and water. These nutrients serve very specific functions that will fail if the body is not properly nourished.

Naturally, if you overnourish your body, it becomes fat and sluggish; if you undernourish it, it gets skinny and weak. In the same way, if your nutritional program is out of balance because you eat too much protein, too many carbohydrates, or too much fat, your body will also suffer. Usually you get fat.

Research shows that 58 percent of American women try to compensate for dietary imbalances by subjecting their bodies to even greater imbalances: crash diets.

CRASH DIETS DON'T WORK

There is no need to starve yourself to lose weight. In fact, starving doesn't work. Your body adapts to a reduced caloric intake by slowing down its metabolism, thus enabling it to survive on increasingly fewer calories. By combining exercise and weight training with sound nutrition, however, you should be able to speed up your metabolism and lose weight on a well-balanced, healthy food program.

We firmly believe that anything below 1200 calories a day for women and 1500 calories for men is borderline starvation. First, on diets of 1000 calories per day or less, your body begins to burn muscle, not fat. Diminishing your protein store causes you to lose muscle mass, which is why so many women look flabby after losing weight on crash diets. We always tell our patients that it's better to be slightly overweight than to starve yourself and lose muscle and skin tone.

Second, while low-calorie diets produce immediate weight loss of up to 5 pounds or more in 3 days, only a small fraction of that loss is body fat. Your first week's weight loss on a low-calorie diet is usually more than 70 percent water.

Third, as we've emphasized before, your body interprets severe caloric reductions as a threat to life, and marshalls all its defenses to ward off this attack. Fat cells actually show biochemical changes as they struggle to maintain size and composition. This results in reduced production of the hormones and enzymes needed for energy production and digestion. Because it is built to survive, the body will slow its metabolism anywhere from 10 to 45 percent within a matter of days. Slower metabolism means fewer calories burned. This means in turn that your body needs to consume fewer calories merely to maintain its current weight. The slowing down of metabolism is a little like turning down the thermostat in your home. The necessary activities continue, but they use less fuel.

A slower metabolism also makes it easier to regain weight on fewer calories than it took to maintain your weight before you began to diet. And because your body does its best to preserve its fat storage cells while you are dieting, it learns to increase its ability to conserve fat. That means not only that you will probably regain weight after a crash diet, but that a higher proportion of your regained pounds are likely to be fat. For instance, if you weighed 200 pounds, with a 40 percent body-fat content, before you dieted, lost 30 pounds on a 900-calorie crash diet, and then resumed a 1880- to 2000-calorie maintenance diet, within a month or two you would have zoomed back up past 200 pounds to 210, with a 45 percent body-fat content! Are those the results you want from a "diet"? Of course not! Your ultimate goal is not just to lose weight, but to lose *fat* weight.

Never go on a reduced-calorie diet unless you also increase your activity level to compensate for your body's automatic metabolic slowdown. All of the women in this book followed food plans of at least 1200 calories per day. This gave them energy for their training sessions, which in turn kept their metabolism humming and allowed them to continue to lose weight.

So many of the women we see in our practice have spent years on a roller coaster of dieting; their weight zooms up and down as they ricochet from one crash diet to another. These women are either robbing their bodies of the nutrients needed for health and vigor, or else overloading their digestive systems with more food than they can properly digest. Either extreme results in depleted energy, lowered immunity, and loss of health and fitness.

Most people on diets have the mistaken impression that all they need to consider is the number of calories consumed per day. They're only half right. The total number of calories is important, but equally significant are the *kind* of calories consumed, and the *source* of those calories. Of course we're talking about junk food here—all the processed, sugared, and fatted goo that translates into saddlebags and bulging tummies. You can't consume a steady diet of junk and be healthy. But there are subtler culprits, too. For example, dairy products are high in calories, fat, and protein. However, most adults don't need dairy products, so their bodies turn those calories into excess body fat. Usually it is stored as a layer of subcutaneous fat that blankets the body and hides muscle definition. That's why we stress a simple and natural, but healthful and satisfying, approach to nutrition. The foods we eat fall into one of three categories: protein, carbohydrates, or fats. Your body needs all three to function properly.

A balanced program of wholesome nutrition, weight training, and exercise produced the impressive changes in the women you met in Chapter 2 of this book. And that combination can produce equally exciting results for you.

PROTEIN

Your body must have protein, which is the basic building block for bones, teeth, and all living cells. It is also needed for tissue repair and replacement, immunity to disease, blood clotting, and the maintenance of the body's essential hormones and secretions. Dietary proteins supply the amino acids required for many metabolic functions. Because there's a constant turnover of protein, it must be constantly replenished.

Each gram of protein supplies the body with 4 calories. The average woman needs about 1 gram of protein for every 2.2 pounds (1 kilogram) of body weigh. If you weight 120 pounds, for example, you should consume about 60 grams of protein a day to maintain your weight. That's equivalent to 1 egg, 3 ounces of fish, and 4 ounces of chicken each day.

Eggs, meat, fish, chicken, soy products, natural cheese and other dairy products, and raw seeds and nuts are all good sources of protein. Since 50–75 percent of the adult population shows an allergic reaction to dairy products, we do not recommend cheese and other dairy products as sources of protein. We avoid milk products.

Proteins are subdivided into two categories: complete and incomplete proteins. Complete proteins are those that come from animals: fish, poultry, or red meat (soybeans, containing a complete vegetable protein, are the only exception). These include all of the essential amino acids. Incomplete proteins come from plants and do not supply the body with all of the amino acids. Many vegetarians who think they are getting sufficient protein supply from legumes, nuts, and seeds are robbing their bodies of essential amino acids. Although it is possible to plan a well-balanced vegetarian diet, it takes a great deal of thought and knowledge, and should be developed by a professional nutritionist. (One other word of caution about vegetarian food plans: We have noticed in our practice that vegetarians who eat so many carbohydrates derived from fruits and vegetables tend to gain excessive amounts of fat around the mid-section. So even though they are low in calories, beware of "bulking up" with carbohydrates.)

We don't like to eat anything artificial—that means anything that's canned, preserved, packaged, etc. Protein powders are included in that category. We feel that they are of low biological value and should be used only in very unusual circumstances. Rather than trying to supplement your diet with protein powder, increase your intake of complete proteins in their natural form.

CARBOHYDRATES

Carbohydrates are probably the most misunderstood of all nutrients. The developers of many crash diets have downplayed the importance of the carbohydrates, leading many people to think that they can eliminate or severely limit their carb intake without hurting their body. That's a great misconception.

Carbohydrates provide the body with immediate energy, and if they are absent, the body automatically makes up for the deficiency. Unfortunately it has no choice but to break down tissue protein for its necessary energy. Also, when the carbohydrate intake is drastically reduced, fats are not completely utilized. When this happens, ketones are produced and the body goes into a state of metabolic imbalance called "ketosis." Serious health problems can result from prolonged ketosis. For good health, the average woman should include at least 100 grams of carbohydrates in her daily diet.

The main function of carbohydrates is to supply fuel for the brain and energy for the body. These nutrients are converted to glucose or stored as glycogen in the liver and muscles, or converted to fat stored as excess adipose tissue. In a well-balanced reducing diet, the body will first use the glucose for immediate energy, then the glycogen, and finally the stored fat. That's the calorie-burning process working at its best.

While we generally think of bread, cereal, pasta, and other grain products as good sources of carbohydrates, the very best sources are fruits and vegetables. They provide bulk in the form of fiber, which helps regulate the elimination process. These foods provide energy to the body during digestion. Refined carbohydrates, such as white flour, and simple carbohydrates, such as sugar and honey, do not provide fiber and are quickly digested, so the glucose gets into the blood stream almost immediately. This not only results in a "sugar high," but increases the appetite. It also causes a rapid drop in blood sugar, so that the body craves more sugar.

Because complex and unrefined carbohydrates have bulk and fiber, they can actually help us lose weight while providing necessary nutrients and satisfying hunger. Like protein, carbohydrates provide 4 calories per gram. Most women need *at the very least* 400 calories of carbohydrates per day.

FATS

Fat also supplies heat and energy, but in a slower-burning form. Except for red blood cells and the cells of the central nervous system, all of the cells in the body can use fatty acids as energy sources. Even the brain can use fatty-acid ketones as energy during a fasting period. Because fats provide 9 calories per gram, they are the body's greatest energy source. But because it's very easy to overindulge in fats, these calorie-rich nutrients are also the greatest cause of bulges.

Fats keep your skin supple and your hair shiny, and facilitate many of your body's functions. Fats help satisfy your appetite and serve as a carrier for the fat-soluble vitamins A, D, E, and K, aiding their absorption in the intestine.

Only minute amounts of this nutrient, however, are necessary for good health. Your body needs no more than 1 tablespoon of fat each day for protein metabolism, to maintain body temperature, and to keep the body functioning properly. Dairy products, avocados, fish, red meat, poultry, butter and margarine, oils, and nuts and nut butters all contain fat, so it's easy to get an oversupply.

In addition to adding extra padding to your body, excessive fats in the diet can be extremely harmful to the heart and vascular system, so we recommend that you use them in moderation. A battle has been raging over the value of polyunsaturated versus saturated fats. Saturated fats are generally those found in meat, dairy products, and chocolate, while the unsaturated kind come mostly from foods of vegetable origin. (Naturally, there are exceptions to this as to every rule: Palm and coconut oil are extremely high in saturated fats, while cod-liver oil contains a high level of polyunsaturates.) Although it has been demonstrated that cholesterol levels increase when saturated fats are ingested, eating too many polyunsaturated fats can also cause problems. They can increase the risk of blood clotting and of gallstones, and may have a negative effect on the heart muscle itself. For these reasons we emphasize that *all* fat in the diet should be kept to a minimum—that is, no more than 200 calories a day.

VITAMINS AND MINERALS

Your body needs both vitamins and minerals to function properly, resist disease and infection, and counteract the effects of too much stress. Vitamins and minerals are nutrients that occur naturally in organic food substances. Eating a well-balanced diet high in natural raw foods is probably the best insurance for most of us, but because many of the fruits and vegetables we eat are grown in soils depleted of minerals and because many of the other foods available have been treated with chemicals, hormones, and other substances that destroy their natural goodness, we also suggest that everyone take some type of vitamin and mineral supplement.

However, before deciding to take any type of dietary supplement, you should have a complete blood study, a nutritional analysis of your diet, and perhaps a hair mineral analysis to determine exactly which deficiencies you may have. You may find that by increasing your intake of natural foods that are high in certain nutrients, your particular deficiencies can be controlled. Food allergy tests have shown, too, that many people are allergic to yeast, corn, and wheat, the foods from which many vitamin supplements are derived. When a person is allergic to these foods, she does not receive the full benefit of the supplement. Hypo-allergenic vitamin supplements are now readily available.

If you are in doubt as to your needs, a multiple vitamin and mineral supplement is usually a good choice. These supplements are formulated by biochemists and are usually well balanced.

SUGGESTED DAILY INTAKE	AVERAGE	DURING HEAVY TRAINING
Vitamin A	10,000 IU	25,000 IU
Vitamin D	400 IU	400 IU
Vitamin C	1,000 IU	2,000 IU
Vitamin E	800 IU	1,000 IU
Vitamin B-1	100 mg	150 mg
Vitamin B-2	100 mg	150 mg
Vitamin B-6	200 mg	250 mg
Vitamin B-12	300 mcg	300 mcg
Niacin or niacinamide	100 mg	200 mg
Pantothenic acid	100 mg	300 mg
Para-amino-benzoic acid	75 mg	250 mg
Choline	100 mg	200 mg
Inositol	100 mg	200 mg
Folic acid	400 mcg	400 mcg
Biotin	100 mcg	100 mcg
Calcium	1,000 mg	2,000 mg
Magnesium	800 mg	1,500 mg
Potassium	200 mg	500 mg
Phosphorus	150 mg	150 mg
Iron	20 mg	20 mg
Iodine	20 mg	20 mg
Copper	2 mg	2 mg
Zinc	25 mg	50 mg
Manganese	20 mg	50 mg
Chromium	750 mg	750 mg
Selenium	100 mcg	100 mcg
Beatine HCl	100 mg	200 mg

(Continued on next page.)

SUGGESTED DAILY INTAKE	AVERAGE	DURING HEAVY TRAINING
Pepsin	50 mg	100 mg
Bromelain	50 mg	50 mg
Ox bile	30 mg	30 mg
Pancreas substance	100 mg	200 mg
Papain	50 mg	100 mg
Protease	100 mg	300 mg
Amylase	25 mg	50 mg
Lipase	25 mg	50 mg

The above chart is only a guideline. If you cannot find the exact amounts of each nutrient listed, then get whatever is closest.

AMINO ACIDS

Once proteins enter the body, they are broken down again into amino acids and nitrogen. These elements are the building blocks of the protein substances created in the body such as hormones, enzymes, and new tissue. In addition, the amino acids aid in the production of bile in the liver, they help control allergic reactions, stimulate fatty acid synthesis, raise the energy level, and even improve the duration and quality of sleep: A number of tests have shown that taking the amino acid tryptophan has greatly helped insomniacs.

There are 22 amino acids, but only 9 are naturally synthesized by our bodies. These are known as the essential amino acids: arginine, histidine (essential for infants only), isoleucine, leucine, lysine, methionine, phenylalanine, threonine, tryptophan, and valine. Together with nitrogen, these amino acids form many different proteins. The nonessential amino acids are: alanine, asparagine, aspartic acid, cysteine, cystine, glutamic acid, glutamine, glycine, hydroxyproline, proline, serine, and tyrosine.

As we noted in the section on protein, many vegetable sources of protein are incomplete. That is, they don't contain enough of the essential amino acids, including lysine, methionine, tryptophan, and threonine. Meat, fish, eggs, and dairy products provide a balance of all the essentials, but eggs are the superior source. The egg's content of amino acids and its balance of these elements is considered to be perfect. Most nutritionists feel that it meets the human body's requirements completely. In fact, when scientists score a food's amino acid content, they judge it against an egg, which is scored at 100. (In addition to providing the essential amino acids, the egg itself supplies the body with 7 grams of pure protein; 3 grams in the yolk and 4 in the white. The yolk contains the fat and most of the egg's 70 calories, so we recommend that fat-conscious eaters make omelettes with 1 whole egg and 2 almost calorie-free whites. It's nourishing, low calorie, and high in amino acids and protein.)

Augmenting the body's intake of amino acids has been a popular practice in weight-training circles for years. Many weight-trained athletes take supplements of arginine and its derivative, ornithine, which aid in muscle growth and the fat-burning process.

As yet, the recommended daily dietary requirements for essential amino acids have not been established; much of the work concerning amino acids is still at the experimental stage. Research is being done to study the relationship between amino acids and weight loss.

We have found that taking amino acid supplements is an excellent way to fortify the diet when calorie intake is restricted. They assist in stabilizing the blood sugar and are great to use in place of sweet snacks when the munchies hit—usually about 11 A.M. and 4 P.M.

GLANDULAR SUPPLEMENTS

During times of stress, the endocrine system, which includes seven glands (the pituitary, thyroid, parathyroid, pancreas, adrenal, ovaries or testes, and pineal) is overworked. Endocrine glands secrete hormones. These glands must work in balance with the nervous system to allow the body to function properly.

Taking glandular supplements can be very beneficial, particularly when the body is under stress, because these glands can quickly become depleted of their hormones. These supplements contain concentrated enzymes and proteins, which provide nutritional value beyond that of vitamins, minerals, and amino acids. However, we do not recommend taking them without a complete examination, including blood tests, hair mineral analysis, and a thorough medical history.

REDESIGN YOUR DIET AS YOU REDESIGN YOUR BODY

The women who redesigned their bodies in Chapter 2 didn't go on crash diets. It was exercise that made the greatest difference for them. But healthy nutrition kept them happy and strong and helped them lose those extra pounds.

They all ate well-balanced meals that totalled about 1200 calories a day. They eliminated dairy products and sugar from their diets and greatly reduced their intake of fats. None of them ever complained of deprivation—in fact, they were so pleased with their new bodies that they reported that giving up milk, sweets, and fatty foods was not only worth it, but easy.

At first the women wanted specific reducing diets, but we gave them a flat "no." If we put them on diets, they'd think of their new way of eating as a temporary phase. We wanted them to consider healthy eating as a new way of life—*forever*. Instead of diets, we showed them how to balance carbohydrates, proteins, and fats in such a way that neither hunger nor weight is a problem. If it sounds too good to be true, take heart: That's what our successful models thought at first too.

The average American woman eats a very poorly balanced diet: 12 to 15 percent protein, 40 to 48 percent fat and 42 to 50 percent carbohydrates. With so much fat in the diet, it's no wonder obesity is one of this country's greatest killers. By simply readjusting those dietary percentages, weight loss and well-being are unavoidable. The optimum diet should be composed as follows:

Protein: 20 percent
Complex carbohydrates: 60–65 percent
Fat: 15–20 percent

In each food category, try to choose items that are the most natural and healthful. Get in the habit of reading labels, and avoid products that contain sugar and additives. For example, when buying bread, look for stone-ground, seven-grain, or pita bread. Natural brown rice is excellent, as are seven-grain cereals. Buy fertile eggs, if possible, and if you must have cheese, choose skim-milk or low-fat varieties. Shop for meat and poultry grown without injected hormones and remove all visible skin or fat before cooking. Try to eat fish and seafoods instead of red meat several times a week, since fish is an excellent source of protein and amino acids, besides being low in fat and calories. For snacks, munch fruits and vegetables; they are excellent sources of vitamins and bulk. Look for pure and natural beverages whenever possible. There's nothing better for you than water or low-sodium mineral water. Pour it over ice with a twist of lemon or lime, and you'll enjoy a healthy, refreshing treat. Herbal teas are also refreshing and cleansing, but try to eliminate coffee and black tea from your diet.

FOODS THAT PROMOTE PROPER NUTRITION:
Spring water
Eggs
Fish
Turkey (skinless breast meat only)
Chicken (skinless breast meat only)
Whole-grain breads and cereals
Fresh vegetables
Fresh fruit

FOODS THAT INHIBIT PROPER NUTRITION:
Processed foods
Dairy products
Sugar
Processed grains (such as white flour, and white rice)
Alcoholic beverages
Black tea
Refined carbohydrates (foods containing white sugar and/or white
    flour such as candy, cakes, cookies, etc.)
Coffee
Salt

It is extremely important to reduce or eliminate added salt from your diet. The human body needs some salt but we almost always get enough from the food we eat. Too much salt can be extremely detrimental to your health. This overused seasoning causes water retention, in addition to contributing to high blood pressure and irritability. Try vegetable seasonings instead. You'll find them just as tasty, and much healthier.

How much hidden sugar and salt do you eat every day? For example, seemingly innocent catsup is more than one-fourth sugar. You probably know that a 12-ounce glass of cola has a shocking 7 teaspoons of sugar, but were you aware that even a stick of chewing gum contains about half a teaspoon? That's a lot. Chicken noodle soup, dill pickles, and soy sauce are foods we think of as harmless, but all are loaded with salt. Even frozen vegetables that list no added salt on the label have been washed in sodium baths before freezing and have a surprisingly high salt content.

Soft drinks, both regular and diet, should be completely eliminated from your diet, whether you're trying to lose, gain, or maintain weight. High in sugar, sodium, and chemicals, regular soft drinks are a hazard to good nutrition. Even worse are the diet versions loaded with artificial sweeteners. Your body doesn't need the sugar, chemicals, or artificial sweeteners, and the excess sodium can actually cause weight gain since it causes the body to retain water and may slow the metabolism. Recent tests have shown that ingredients in a number of condiments such as pepper, mustard, horseradish, and wood-smoke flavorings stimulate the appetite and may be carcinogenic (cancer-causing). Use them sparingly, if at all.

Enjoy your salads and steamed vegetables without dressings. Sprinkle on a little lemon juice or vinegar, and experiment with vegetable seasonings. You'll find yourself enjoying the natural flavor of your foods instead of smothering them with salt. You'll also notice less water retention, and perhaps even lower blood pressure.

While the body needs some fat to fuel the nervous system, to encourage hormone production, and to provide a feeling of satisfied fullness, too much fat in the diet contributes to heart and vascular problems. If you're overweight, remember that fat has 9 calories per gram, while protein and complex carbohydrates each have only 4 calories per gram, making fats a much more "expensive" way to fill up, calorie-wise.

There are also some simple habits you can acquire to improve your nutrition:

1. Don't eat if you're not hungry.
2. If a food doesn't appeal to you, don't eat it.
3. Stop eating before you are full.
4. Eat only at mealtimes.
5. Eat only when you are sitting at a table.
6. Chew slowly and thoroughly.
7. Reduce distractions (TV, radio, reading, etc.).
8. Eat at least 3 meals a day.
9. Don't skip breakfast—it's the meal that sets your pace for the day.
10. Eat when you are feeling serene—a calm emotional state helps your body to digest food properly.

We recommend that you have protein at each meal—since it takes longer to digest than carbohydrates, it provides sustained energy for up to 4 hours afterwards. Most high-protein food also contains fat, which digests very slowly and also contributes to the full feeling. Carbohydrates, on the other hand, provide energy for less than 2 hours. That's why a breakfast of cereal and fruit doesn't keep you satisfied as long one with eggs does. That's why you're hungry just a short while after a lunch at the salad bar. Complex carbohydrates should be eaten along with protein, allowing the protein to be used for tissue building, while the carbs provide the body with its necessary energy. Increased carbohydrate intake will also help fat to metabolize faster and perform its necessary work rather than turning into excess body fat.

We also suggest that when selecting protein foods, you should choose low-fat proteins. Fish has the lowest percentage of fat, while chicken and turkey breast (without the skin!) come next. Red meat, even the lean variety, has an exceptionally high fat content, and dairy products have the most. A 2-ounce piece of cheese has more fat than a 4-ounce steak. Eggs also contain fat and cholesterol, but because the egg is rich with choline and lecithin, these fats break down rapidly into energy and are more completely utilized than fats from dairy products.

In addition, be sure to drink at least 6 to 8 glasses of water each day. Many women restrict their water intake, thinking that the more they drink, the more they retain. But just the opposite is true. When you limit your water consumption, your body begins to conserve the fluid it has in order to protect itself against dehydration. By drinking less water, you are actually training your body to hold onto what it has. It needs water to flush away waste and rid itself of the toxins that are often unavoidable in daily life. Too little water can also hasten premature aging of the skin.

When you eat can be almost as important as *what* you eat. It's a well-known fact that high-calorie foods are burned off more efficiently during the day than at night. Try having 3 ounces of protein for breakfast and dinner, with the larger serving of 4 ounces at lunch. And consume fats in the early part of the day, too. Because of their high calorie content, eating controlled amounts of fats earlier in the day will keep you satisfied on less food.

Also consider what day you eat a given food. We firmly believe that rotating your food intake is a key to healthy nutrition and weight loss. We suggest that no food should be consumed more often than once in 4 days. In this way you are forced to eat a greater variety of foods and will have more opportunity to consume all of the nutrients your body needs. Many people too have allergic reactions to certain foods. By rotating foods, it becomes much easier to tell which ones upset your body and which promote your best health. By keeping a daily food diary in which you write down everything you eat, you'll gradually learn the patterns of your eating, and which foods cause negative reactions. It's a wonderful tool.

FOOD ALLERGIES

You are probably allergic to a variety of foods and don't even know it. Food allergies don't always manifest themselves by producing skin rashes and hives. Experts say that from 60 to 80 percent of adults have allergies that are undetected because they produce such symptoms as headache, fatigue, sinusitis, ear and throat infections, symptoms which are usually attributed to other causes. Food allergies can also inhibit digestion, increase water retention and even retard weight loss. Some people experience restlessness, depression and insatiable hunger leading to binge eating after they eat foods to which they are allergic.

And, just as a smoker craves nicotine and an alcoholic longs for a drink, we are often addicted to the very substances to which we have allergies. We consume more and more of the offending foods, thus becoming even more addicted and suffering even greater discomfort, without realizing the cause of the problem. Milk is a leading source of food allergies, but so are chocolate, cola, corn, and citrus fruits and vegetables. Eggs, legumes, tomatoes and wheat are also frequent culprits.

How can you tell which foods you're allergic to, realizing that they're probably things you eat everyday? We feel that the most accurate way to detect hidden allergies is through cytotoxic blood tests, in which a small amount of your blood is tested for compatibility with hundreds of different foods, vitamins, minerals and chemical additives.

The accuracy of this test is between 60 and 80 per cent, depending on the clinic that performs the test. The test measures the reaction of the white blood cells in your blood stream to those various substances. Allergy-producing foods are those which cause white blood cells to change shape or even rupture in this laboratory procedure, indicating a violent reaction to the offending substance. White blood cells make up a big part of the body's immune system and help to fight off toxins. If they're busy defending against toxic foods, they don't do a complete job protecting the system from bacteria, viruses and other harmful agents. That means your resistance is low.

These tests are still not readily available in many parts of the country. By carefully monitoring what you put into your body, you will soon become keenly aware of how your body reacts to various foods. You must begin to listen to your body, to get in touch with what foods help and which hinder your feeling of health and well-being. You are going to be the best judge of what foods should or shouldn't go into your mouth.

But there's another, simpler way to check for blatant allergies and it doesn't cost a cent. Check your pulse 20 to 30 minutes after eating a particular food that you suspect might be an allergen. If your pulse rate stays the same or increases less than 10 beats per minute, the food is non-toxic or low stress. But if there is a sharp rise, your body is telling you that the food is producing a definite allergic reaction. Again, not all medical authorities agree on the effectiveness of this test.

NOTE: In our chiropractic office, we also use muscle-testing procedures which indicate food allergies.

LOW FAT, LOW ALLERGY, QUICK WEIGHT LOSS ROTATION FOOD PROGRAM

Shown here is a food program we have put together for you to use as an example. We call it our Low Fat, Low Allergy, Quick Weight Loss Rotation Food Program. By looking at the way in which we rotated foods in a four-day cycle, you can develop a program of your own which we hope will incorporate a similarly wide variety of foods. The menu below is *just a sample* of the many different foods you can eat while on a food-rotation program.

The program stabilizes blood sugar, reduces allergic reactions, and induces quick weight loss. It is also extremely well balanced, providing complex carbohydrates, protein, and a small amount of fat at each meal.

Processed sugar is poison to your body, and has been eliminated from this diet. Without this appetite stimulant, you'll quickly find yourself losing your craving for sweets.

Alcohol has also been eliminated, because of its empty calories and tendency to promote water retention.

We have also eliminated foods found to produce allergies in a high percentage of adults. For example, the program contains no milk or other dairy products, since they have caused allergic reactions among so many people who have undergone food-allergy tests.

If you think you might have hidden allergies, we suggest that you try a food-rotation program for 12 weeks, repeating the 4-day rotation. As you become more sensitive to your body and its responses, you can probably begin to pinpoint which foods are harmful to you, and eliminate them from your diet.

FOUR-DAY SAMPLE MENU

Day 1:
Breakfast

½ fresh grapefruit
1 slice whole wheat toast
1 egg

Lunch

4 oz. filet of sole (broiled dry)
1 cup green beans
1 small mixed green salad:
    Lettuce
    Red cabbage
    Vinegar or lemon dressing with herb seasoning
Water, mineral water (low sodium), coffee, tea
Pineapple slices, 3 oz.

Dinner

1 cup steamed asparagus
4 oz. veal
1 small baked potato
½ cup grapes

BEVERAGES: Water, mineral water (low sodium), coffee, tea. Drink at least 6 glasses of water; limit coffee and tea to 2 cups daily. These beverages are suitable for each day's menu.

SNACKS: Raw cauliflower, jicama, anise

Day 2:
Breakfast

½ papaya
2 oz. rye flakes with ½ teaspoon tupelo honey

Lunch

3½ oz. tuna, water-packed albacore
½ hardtack rye cracker
4 oz. alfalfa sprouts
Mustard
1 cup strawberries

Dinner

Salad made from ¼ small avocado and ½ cup sliced mushrooms, tossed with vinegar
4 oz. liver (sautéed)
½ cup onions
1 cup brussels sprouts
½ cup cherries or 2 plums

SNACKS: Frozen watermelon pops available from health food stores. (Check package to see that they contain 50 calories or less.)

Day 3:
Breakfast

1 medium pear
4 oz. tofu
Cinnamon
1 rice cake, unsalted

Lunch

4 oz. chicken breast, broiled with herbs
4 oz. peas
1 cup watercress salad
1 tangerine, 4 oz.

Dinner

4 oz. halibut, broiled dry with herbs
½ cup brown rice
1 cup cooked carrots
1 kiwi fruit, medium

Day 4:
Breakfast

1 medium orange
2 oz. oat flakes, cooked, sprinkled with raisins and
sunflower seeds

Lunch

Turkey tostada:
Corn tortilla, warmed in oven (crisp) and topped with
   4 oz. turkey breast
   Shredded cabbage
   Radishes
   Tomato
   Zucchini
   1 oz. chili sauce (no preservatives)
1 medium peach

Dinner

4 oz. perch, broiled dry with herbs
1 cup steamed spinach
1 medium apple

SNACKS: Air-popped popcorn, 2 cups, no butter. May season with herbs and spices.

*WE RECOMMEND THAT NUTRITIONAL SUPPLEMENTS BE TAKEN WITH MEALS.

EXERCISE INDEX

WEIGHT AND EXERCISE RECORDS

WEIGHT AND EXERCISE RECORDS

WEIGHT AND EXERCISE RECORDS

WEIGHT AND EXERCISE RECORDS